T0202337

Acute and Critical Care Echocardiography

Acute and Critical Care Echocardiography

Edited by

Claire Colebourn

Consultant Medical Intensivist, John Radcliffe Hospital, Oxford, UK

Jim Newton

Consultant Cardiologist, John Radcliffe Hospital, Oxford, UK

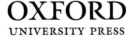

OXFORD

UNIVERSITY PRESS

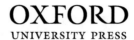

OXFORD

UNIVERSITY PRESS

Great Clarendon Street, Oxford, OX2 6DP,
United Kingdom

Oxford University Press is a department of the University of Oxford.
It furthers the University's objective of excellence in research, scholarship,
and education by publishing worldwide. Oxford is a registered trade mark of
Oxford University Press in the UK and in certain other countries

© Oxford University Press 2017

The moral rights of the authors have been asserted

First Edition published in 2017

All rights reserved. No part of this publication may be reproduced, stored in
a retrieval system, or transmitted, in any form or by any means, without the
prior permission in writing of Oxford University Press, or as expressly permitted
by law, by licence or under terms agreed with the appropriate reprographics
rights organization. Enquiries concerning reproduction outside the scope of the
above should be sent to the Rights Department, Oxford University Press, at the
address above

You must not circulate this work in any other form
and you must impose this same condition on any acquirer

Published in the United States of America by Oxford University Press
198 Madison Avenue, New York, NY 10016, United States of America

British Library Cataloguing in Publication Data

Data available

Library of Congress Control Number: 2017936919

ISBN 978–0–19–875716–0

Printed and bound in Great Britain by
CPI Group (UK) Ltd, Croydon, CR0 4YY

Oxford University Press makes no representation, express or implied, that the
drug dosages in this book are correct. Readers must therefore always check
the product information and clinical procedures with the most up-to-date
published product information and data sheets provided by the manufacturers
and the most recent codes of conduct and safety regulations. The authors and
the publishers do not accept responsibility or legal liability for any errors in the
text or for the misuse or misapplication of material in this work. Except where
otherwise stated, drug dosages and recommendations are for the non-pregnant
adult who is not breast-feeding

Links to third party websites are provided by Oxford in good faith and
for information only. Oxford disclaims any responsibility for the materials
contained in any third party website referenced in this work.

Foreword

Echocardiography is the first line technique for the detection and evaluation of abnormal cardiac structure and function. Historically this has been performed according to a standardized protocol of views by specialist clinical scientists, cardiologists or radiographers. In the last 10 years, the concept of a point-of-care study using the ultrasound machine as an 'ultrasonic stethoscope' has evolved. These studies are not full echocardiograms but rather an extension of the clinical examination. These allow the immediate detection of major pathology potentially requiring emergency life-saving treatment. Some acute medicine or intensive care specialists will want to restrict themselves to point-of-care studies but many will enlarge their experience to become expert at assessments not traditionally part of cardiology-based echocardiography departments. These include the effects of blunt or open trauma, and sepsis but also response to filling or the effects of different regimes of mechanical ventilation or the assessment of extracorporeal circulations. This book is an excellent summary of cardiac ultrasound in acute and critical care and will guide initial training and act as an aide-memoire for the more experienced practitioner. It is well-laid out, clearly written, and pragmatic. I thoroughly recommend it.

John Chambers
Professor of Clinical Cardiology Guy's and St Thomas' Hospitals
Past-President of the British Society of Echocardiography

Preface

Over the last decade, the subspecialty of critical care echocardiography has been recognized, shaped, and formalized by the British Society of Echocardiography. Locally, we have joined this process with the development of the Oxford Critical Care Echo Fellowship. The Fellowship was set up in 2009 and, to date, has provided training for six specialist critical care trainees, each of whom have authored chapters relevant to their area of specialist interest.

This book is designed to give you a comprehensive understanding of the assessment of all aspects of cardiac structure and function, with specific reference to patients who require organ support. We have used case studies with still and moving images throughout the text. The case studies come from our experience over the last 7 years of using transthoracic echocardiography to guide patient care in a tertiary intensive care unit admitting over 1000 patients annually. The cases address questions commonly asked of critical care echocardiographers and explain how echo findings can be used to influence management, interventions, and hopefully outcome.

Much like critical care echocardiography, this book has been a joint effort between critical care and cardiology, and we hope you find it easy to use and useful in the care of your critically ill patients.

If you would like to contact us about service delivery, training issues, or interesting clinical scenarios, we would be delighted to hear from you.

CC and JN

Contents

Abbreviations

A4C	apical four-chamber (view)	g	gram
A&E	accident and emergency	Hb	haemoglobin
ACCE	Adult Critical Care Echocardiography	HFNEF	heart failure with a normal ejection fraction
ACE	angiotensin-converting enzyme	ICE-BLU	Intensive Care Echo–Basic Lung Ultrasound
AF	atrial fibrillation		
AKI	acute kidney injury	ICS	Intensive Care Society
AMP	adenosine monophosphate	IE	infective endocarditis
aMVL	anterior mitral valve leaflet	IMR	ischaemic mitral regurgitation
APD	anterior–posterior distance	INR	international normalized ratio
AR	aortic regurgitation	IVC	inferior vena cava
AS	aortic stenosis	J	joule
ASD	atrial septal defect	JA	jet area
AT	acceleration time	kg	kilogram
ATP	adenosine triphosphate	kPa	kilopascal
AVI	atrioventricular interdependence	LA	left atrium
BMV	balloon mitral valvotomy	LV	left ventricle
bpm	beat per minute	LVEDP	left ventricular end-diastolic pressure
BSA	body surface area	LVH	left ventricular hypertrophy
BSE	British Society of Echocardiography	LVOT	left ventricular outflow tract
CK	creatine kinase	m	metre
cm	centimetre	MAP	mean arterial pressure
cmH_2O	centimetre of water	MAPSE	mitral annulus plane systolic excursion
COX-2	cyclo-oxygenase 2	mg	milligram
CPAP	continuous positive airways pressure	MI	myocardial infarction
CRP	C-reactive protein	min	minute
CT	computed tomography	ml	millilitre
CTPA	computed tomography pulmonary angiography	mm	millimetre
		mmHg	millimetre of mercury
CW	continuous wave	mmol	millimole
2D	two-dimensional	MPI	myocardial performance index
3D	three-dimensional	MR	mitral regurgitation
dL	decilitre	MRI	magnetic resonance imaging
ECG	electrocardiogram	mRNA	messenger ribonucleic acid
EF	ejection fraction	ms	millisecond
EI	eccentricity index	MS	mitral stenosis
EROA	effective regurgitant orifice area	MV	mitral valve
FAC	fractional area change	MVA	mitral valve area
FICE	Focused Intensive Care Echocardiography	MVP	mitral valve leaflet prolapse
		NIV	non-invasive ventilation
FiO_2	inspired oxygen concentration	OSCE	Objective Structured Clinical Examination
FS	fractional shortening		

$P_{1/2}$	pressure half-time	RVEF	right ventricular ejection fraction
PA	pulmonary artery	RVFAC	right ventricular fractional area change
$PaCO_2$	partial pressure of carbon dioxide	RVOT	right ventricular outflow tract
PADP	pulmonary artery diastolic pressure	RVSP	right ventricular systolic pressure
PAP	pulmonary artery pressure	s	second
PASP	pulmonary artery systolic pressure	SAM	systolic anterior motion
PAT	pulmonary acceleration time	SBT	spontaneous breathing trial
PE	pulmonary embolism	SV	stroke volume
PEEP	positive end-expiratory pressure	SVR	systemic vascular resistance
PHT	pulmonary hypertension	SVV	stroke volume variation
PISA	proximal isovelocity surface area	TAPSE	tricuspid annular plane systolic excursion
PLAX	parasternal long axis		
PM	papillary muscle	TDi	tissue Doppler imaging
pMVL	posterior mitral valve leaflet	TOE	transoesophageal echocardiography
PP	pericardial pressure	TR	tricuspid regurgitation
PR	pulmonary regurgitation	TTE	transthoracic echocardiography
PRIS	propofol-related infusion syndrome	UK	United Kingdom
PVR	pulmonary vascular resistance	VC	vena contracta
RAP	right atrial pressure	vs	versus
RF	rheumatic fever	VTE	venous thromboembolism
RV	right ventricle	VTI	velocity time integral
RVEDP	right ventricular end-diastolic pressure	WCC	white cell count

Contributors

Graham Barker Consultant in Intensive Care and Anaesthetics, John Radcliffe Hospital, Oxford, UK *Chapter 2*

Claire Colebourn Consultant Medical Intensivist, John Radcliffe Hospital, Oxford, UK *Chapters 1 and 8*

James Day Senior Registrar in Intensive Care and Anaesthetics, John Radcliffe Hospital, Oxford, UK *Chapter 4*

David Garry Consultant in Intensive Care and Anaesthetics, John Radcliffe Hospital, Oxford, UK *Chapter 3*

Justin Mandeville Consultant in Intensive Care and Anaesthetics, Stoke Mandeville Hospital, Buckinghamshire, UK *Chapters 6 and 7*

Jim Newton Consultant Cardiologist, John Radcliffe Hospital, Oxford, UK *Chapter 5*

Jodie Smythe Senior Registrar in Intensive Care and Anaesthetics, John Radcliffe Hospital, Oxford, UK *Chapter 5*

Toby Thomas Consultant in Intensive Care and Anaesthetics, National Hospital for Neurology and Neurosurgery, London, UK *Chapter 5*

Digital media accompanying the book

Individual purchasers of this book are entitled to free personal access to accompanying digital media in the online edition. Please refer to the access token card for instructions on token redemption and access.

These online ancillary materials, where available, are noted with iconography throughout the book.

There are over 80 videos of transthoracic echocardiography. These show assessment of aspects of cardiac structure and function encountered in critically unwell patients. Cases demonstrate the views you can expect to see and how to interpret these to inform management, interventions, and hopefully outcome.

The corresponding media can be found on *Oxford Medicine Online* at: http://www.oxford-medicine.com/acutecriticalecho.

If you are interested in access to the complete online edition, please consult with your librarian.

The subspecialty practice of critical care echocardiography

Transthoracic echocardiography (TTE) has become a unique tool with which to care for the critically unwell patient. The non-invasive nature of this imaging modality, coupled with rapid recent technical development providing high-quality scanning at the bedside, fits contemporary critical care practice.

The last 20 years of critical care research has directed us away from blood pressure and cardiac output targets and towards achieving an understanding of the circulation on a case-by-case basis and directing therapy towards achieving adequate organ perfusion. Never before has it been so relevant to clinicians in critical care to have a working knowledge of individual cardiac structure and function on which to base clinical decision-making.

Over the decade between 2000 and 2010, a growing awareness of the potential use of non-invasive imaging in critical illness generated pockets of enthusiastic, and often expert, practice, but without regulation or guidance from a governing body.

Although, in 2009, a statement was released encouraging the use and attempted regulation of critical care echocardiography, it took another three years before a regulating committee was set up through joint working between the British Society of Echocardiography (BSE) and the Intensive Care Society (ICS).

This committee designed and published two separate processes for the acquisition of critical care echocardiography skills:

- Focused Intensive Care Echocardiography (FICE): a first responder scan designed to be used for all patients needing critical care input whether within or outside the intensive care unit. Responsibility for FICE certification now rests with the ICS.

- Adult Critical Care Echocardiography (ACCE): a full echocardiographic study providing structural and haemodynamic information in patients requiring critical care input. This examination process now sits alongside the pre-existing Adult Transthoracic and Adult Transoesophageal examination processes run by the BSE as a third distinct area of practice.

FICE and ACCE are undoubtedly linked but are not intended to follow on from one another and cannot be viewed as a two-step process; it is therefore possible to train in critical care echocardiography without achieving FICE accreditation beforehand. FICE accreditation is, however, a good way of getting a flavour of critical care echocardiography in order to make a decision about whether to undertake ACCE accreditation. The lack of an intermediate step between FICE and ACCE was a carefully made decision, safe practice within FICE is based on qualitative assessment. ACCE level practice incorporates both qualitative and quantitative assessment. An intermediate training step would therefore inevitably encourage a set of incomplete quantitative assessments, which risk being incorrect and misinterpreted.

Obtaining and optimizing acoustic windows in critical illness

British accreditation in non-cardiac critical care echocardiography is now based solely upon the transthoracic modality. The decision to take this approach swims against the tide of opinion prevailing at the turn of the millennium, but is concurrent with real-world practice and the evidence base.

The decision to direct critical care echocardiography practice towards the transthoracic approach is based on the following factors:

1. Modern imaging platforms have largely removed concerns about poor imaging quality in the critically ill

2. TTE removes the risk of oesophageal rupture which, although occurs in only 1 in 1000 transoesophageal echocardiograms (TOEs), carries a higher and unnecessary risk in the intubated patient

3. Evidence shows that acoustic windows provide diagnostic information in 95% of unselected critically unwell patients undergoing transthoracic assessment

4. The diagnostic information achieved using TTE changes clinical pathways in approximately 40–50% of patients, making it one of the most clinically effective investigations in critical care practice

5. A large proportion of patients in critical care areas are not intubated, and intubation for airway protection to facilitate a TOE would rarely be in the patient's best interests; this is particularly true of patients we are required to review and manage on the wards and in accident and emergency (A&E) departments

6. Intubation of the oesophagus alters the intrathoracic pressure, removing some of the haemodynamic assessment capabilities of echocardiography

7. By focusing skills on a single modality, we maximize our chances of remaining highly competent and therefore reduce the rate of failure to obtain useful images using the transthoracic approach.

A TOE should be viewed as a separate test with specific indications, including:

- Detailed mitral valve assessment
- Search for posterior aortic root abscesses
- Assessment of valvular destruction and pre-surgical workup in bacterial endocarditis
- Suspicion of aortic dissection above the level of the aortic root.

This approach translates into clinical practice. Our local experience in Oxford, a two-site 24-bedded medical and surgical intensive care unit which also cares for high-dependency patients, is that we perform 600 clinical and training echocardiograms per annum and approximately 10 TOEs are indicated from these studies.

Critically ill patients are undoubtedly amongst the most challenging echo subjects for many of the following reasons:

- Difficulty accessing the patient due to lines and other equipment
- Suboptimal positioning
- Body wall oedema
- Drains and dressings covering imaging areas
- Lung pathology causing interference with imaging during the respiratory cycle.

Many of these factors can be overcome by:

- Spending time and care preparing and positioning the patient: this is crucial in our practice
- Imaging early in the patient's clinical course
- Re-imaging when body wall oedema has reduced
- Using the subcostal window, including modified subcostal views, to obtain long and short axis assessment of the heart.

Figure 1.1 shows a member of our echo team imaging a patient and illustrates the following features of good practice improving safety and efficacy.

- The patient has been carefully turned into the left lateral position to maximize acoustic windows; this is the single most important factor in achieving good transthoracic images
- The lines and filtration set have been directed off the top of the bed to remain out of the echocardiographer's field
- Drains and catheter bags have been carefully moved away from the imaging site
- The bed height has been adjusted to allow easy access for echocardiography

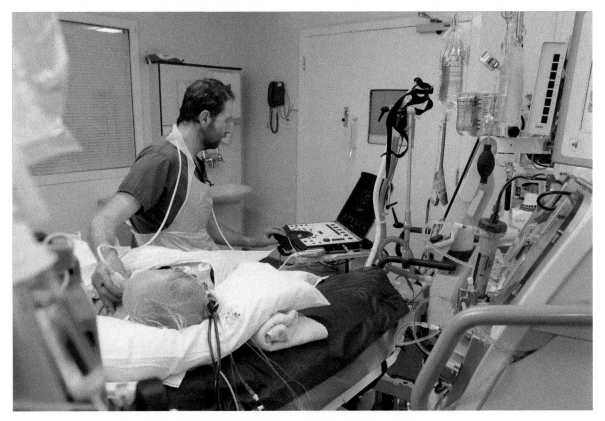

Figure 1.1 **Demonstration of good bedside echo practice to optimize imaging quality.**

- A space has been cleared next to the patient and covered with protective pads to prevent cross-contamination from the procedure

- The ventilator has been positioned away from the echo machine and the endotracheal tube support adjusted to stay out of the echocardiographer's field

- Compact, high-quality portable equipment is being used

- The patient has been placed in a comfortable and supported position, and the bedside nurse or another assistant is local to provide patient support if required.

The patient shown in the photograph had been in the critical care unit for four days on multi-organ support when these images were taken. Figures 1.2 (a) and (b) 📷 and 1.2 (c) demonstrates the diagnostic quality of the echocardiographic images that can be achieved in this setting.

Using echocardiography in the initial stabilization of the critically ill

The FICE protocol

FICE is intended to be used to rapidly assess the critically unwell, and often hypotensive, patient to rule in or rule out pathologies requiring immediate lifesaving treatment.

In line with this concept, the FICE protocol is based on bold qualitative evidence of five cardiac conditions:

1. Cardiac tamponade: requires immediate drainage

2. Gross left ventricular failure: aids decision-making

3. Gross hypovolaemia: requires intravascular filling

4. Acute right heart dysfunction: indicates an acute massive pulmonary embolus where this fits the clinical picture

5. Deep pleural effusion: can cause mediastinal shift and hypovolaemia.

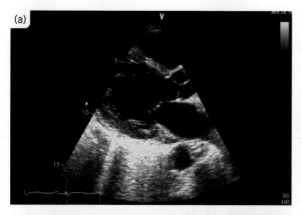

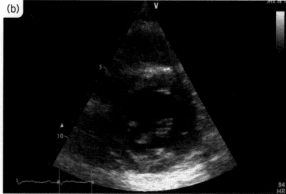

Figures 1.2 (a) [Video 1.1], (b) [Video 1.2], and (c) Images achieved using bedside echocardiography following 4 days of multi-organ support.

🎥 *These videos are available to watch in the online video appendix.*
© Oxford University Hospitals NHS Foundation Trust 2016, with permission.

The FICE protocol employs four cardiac imaging windows and imaging of the pleural spaces to look for evidence of these five clinical scenarios. Where pathology is gross, it may be easily identified from a single image, and treatment should be started as soon as a reasonable conclusion has been reached. Findings should be recorded and archived according to local practices to serve as documentation of findings, so that actions taken based on the images obtained can be evidenced and audited.

The FICE protocol standard views are shown in Table 1.1, with the findings that should be sought for each of the previously described pathologies in those views.

Steps to accreditation

The FICE training process takes place over a six to nine month period. Sign-off is on a minimum of 50 cases; more may be required to achieve competency.

1. Identify a local mentor at registration; a national database of mentors is available on the ICS website.

2. Attend a FICE-approved basic echo course.

3. Perform the initial ten cases directly observed and assisted by a mentor or supervisor.

4. Complete a logbook of 50 studies, with regular review of studies for assessment of quality and judgement; every 7–10 cases should be reviewed or more frequently if there are problems with obtaining images.

5. All studies must be collected within a 12-month period from the first to last scans and the studies must be archived.

6. Perform a 'triggered assessment' echo with your supervisor when you and your mentor think you are ready. The exact number of cases performed prior to this may be greater than 50, depending upon how quickly your skills develop.

Table 1.1 FICE protocol images and key findings according to pathology

View	Tamponade	Acute left ventricular dysfunction	Gross hypovolaemia	Acute right heart dysfunction	Deep pleural effusion
Parasternal long axis	Look for fluid around the LV that comes to a sharp point between the atrium and the descending aorta	Look for poor left ventricular wall movement; the walls should move in to halve the size of the left ventricular cavity in a normally functioning heart	The left ventricular cavity looks small (approximately 3 cm wide) and the walls may touch each other with each cardiac cycle. The RV will appear slit-like and collapsed	The RV should be approximately the size of an apricot in this view. If the diameter is wider than this, suspect right ventricular dilatation	Depth out to reveal fluid that reflects **onto** the left atrium. Beware coexisting pericardial and pleural fluid; ensure your depth is great enough to see both
Parasternal short axis	Fluid may be seen encircling, and even crushing, the LV	Look for minimal change in cavity size with each cardiac cycle	The left ventricular cavity looks small (approximately 3 cm wide) and the walls may touch each other with each cardiac cycle. The RV will appear slit-like and collapsed	The RV should hug the left ventricular wall when not dilated. Look for a right ventricular cavity that is approaching the same size as the LV or larger	Look for fluid around the heart that contains lung
Apical four-chamber	Fluid may be seen encircling, and even crushing, the LV and RV. In a huge pericardial effusion, the heart may appear to swing within the pericardial sac	Look for poor left ventricular wall movement; the walls should move in to halve the size of the left ventricular cavity in a normally functioning heart	The left ventricular cavity looks small (approximately 3 cm wide) and the walls may touch each other with each cardiac cycle. The RV will appear slit-like and collapsed	The RV may appear to be the same size or larger than the LV, and annular vertical movement may appear reduced	Pleural fluid is not well seen in this view
Subcostal	Fluid may be seen encircling, and even crushing, the LV and RV. In a huge pericardial effusion, the heart may appear to swing within the pericardial sac	Look for poor left ventricular wall movement; the walls should move in to halve the size of the left ventricular cavity in a normally functioning heart	The left ventricular cavity looks small. The RV will appear slit-like and collapsed. The IVC is <1.5 cm in diameter and collapses deeply on inspiration	The RV may appear to be the same size or larger than the LV, and annular vertical movement may appear reduced	Pleural fluid is not well seen in this view
Pleural spaces					Locate the hemi-diaphragms and measure the depth of fluid above them. A haemodynamically significant effusion is likely to be 10 cm deep. An effusion affecting oxygenation or work of breathing will be between 5 and 10 cm in depth

IVC, inferior vena cava; LV, left ventricle; RV, right ventricle.

7. The 'Intensive Care Echo–Basic Lung Ultrasound' (ICE-BLU) training module available through the ICS website should also be completed.

8. The summary sign-off sheet and evidence of the completed logbook and online learning module should then be sent to the ICS secretariat.

9. FICE accreditation will then be awarded at the discretion of the Chair of the FICE Committee.

10. Before undertaking FICE accreditation, consider carefully whether you will be able to maintain your skills.

Who can act as a supervisor?

Your supervisor needs accreditation with the BSE in any TTE examination or an equivalent European accreditation.

Who can act as a mentor?

- This is currently less clearly defined but would include:
  - Those with BSE accreditation in adult TTE or ACCE
  - Those working towards the above-mentioned examinations
  - Experienced current FICE practitioners with support from a BSE-accredited supervisor.

The mentor must be able to perform at a sufficient level of expertise to identify mistakes in the interpretation of echo findings and to correct practical technique in a skilled manner.

Further information about FICE accreditation can be found at the following web address: http://www.ics.ac.uk/ICS/fice.aspx.

The current consensus guidelines on the management of circulatory shock by the European Society of Intensive Care Medicine recommend the use of echocardiography where the cause of shock is uncertain or when patients do not respond to initial therapy based on clinical assessment. Use of the FICE protocol in this setting is therefore highly appropriate.

CASE STUDY
Putting the FICE protocol into action

The night intensive care registrar was asked to review a 27-year-old man who had been intubated and ventilated for some weeks due to profound critical illness neuromyopathy following an episode of mesenteric ischaemia. The patient had a persistent sinus tachycardia of over 120 bpm. On clinical examination, he was found to be peripherally vasoconstricted with a systolic blood pressure of 80 mmHg. On review of the patient's clinical parameters, the attending registrar found that this physiology had been developing over a number of days. A FICE scan was performed which demonstrated a deep circumferential loculated pericardial effusion and a moderate-sized pleural effusion. Figure 1.3 🔴 shows the FICE scan findings.

The night registrar contacted a senior member of the critical care echo team to query a diagnosis of cardiac tamponade. They attended the patient and confirmed the diagnosis of cardiac tamponade using more advanced echo techniques. The pericardial space was needle-decompressed with a 10-mmHg rise in systolic blood pressure. The patient was then managed with a thoracoscopic pericardial drainage procedure, with a return of normal haemodynamics the following day.

Further key pathologies that can be detected by the FICE protocol

The FICE protocol can also be used safely to detect:

- Severe left ventricular failure
- Gross hypovolaemia and
- Acute right heart dysfunction.

Examples of how to identify these diagnoses are given in Figures 1.4, 1.5, and 1.6 🔴

Adult Critical Care Echocardiography accreditation

This accreditation process was set up in October 2012 to address the specific needs of the intensive care clinician

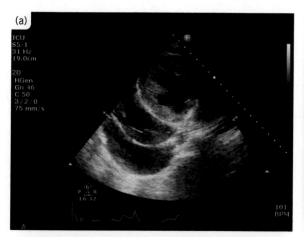

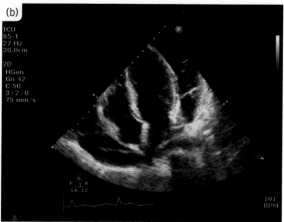

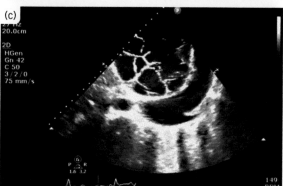

Figure 1.3 (a) [Video 1.3] (b) [Video 1.4], and (c) [Video 1.5] Parasternal long axis, apical four-chamber, and retrocardiac images of a loculated, large-volume pericardial effusion and a moderate-volume, left-sided pleural effusion.

These videos are available to watch in the online video appendix.
© Oxford University Hospitals NHS Foundation Trust 2016, with permission.

wishing to lead echo within their department and practise high-quality echocardiography to address cardiac diagnostics and haemodynamic assessment in their patients.

This accreditation now sits alongside the Adult Transthoracic accreditation and the Adult Trans-oesophageal accreditation as the third adult accreditation process offered and overseen by the BSE.

The syllabus is based around the minimum BSE data set alongside specific features of echo in the critically unwell patient such as the impact of ventilation and the assessment of fluid responsiveness.

The full syllabus can be accessed through the BSE website at the following web address: http://www.bse-cho.org/media/103691/accreditation_pack_-__cc_october_20132.pdf.

The accreditation process has been designed to be achievable by a consultant clinician who has one four hour session allocated to echo training per week over a two year period.

Accreditation

Accreditation requires:

* Logbook collection: 250 echo cases should be performed and reported over a 24-month period which reflect the minimum data set and include a clinically relevant conclusion. Up to 50 of these studies can be repeats, for example re-assessment of fluid responsiveness following initial therapy

* Satisfactory performance in multiple choice question exam: the multiple choice questions reflect essential elements of practice, generic to all forms of echocardiography, for example ultrasound physics and valvular assessment, and specific elements of clinical practice in critical care

* Submission of five demonstration cases and performance of a complete echocardiogram on a normal subject in an examination setting: this is a new Objective Structured Clinical Examination

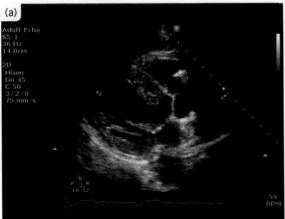

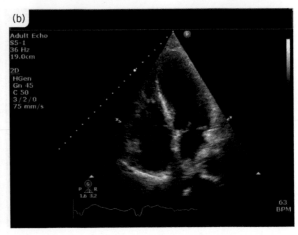

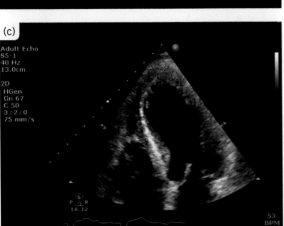

Figure 1.4 (a) [Video 1.6] (b) [Video 1.7], and (c) [Video 1.8] Severe left ventricular failure.

These videos are available to watch in the online video appendix.
© Oxford University Hospitals NHS Foundation Trust 2016, with permission.

(OSCE) initiative being adopted for all BSE accreditation processes.

The OSCE is divided into three stages:

- Review of the candidate's logbook
- Performance of an echo examination on a normal subject, demonstrating correct probe movements and optimization of the images
- Review of demonstration cases which must include:
  - One case illustrating the assessment of fluid responsiveness and one case of assessment of shock from any cause. These cases must be performed in the critical care environment on a patient who is critically unwell
  - One case must be completely normal
  - The remaining two cases are the candidate's choice and, in line with the Transthoracic Accreditation process, should demonstrate

moderate to severe valvular pathology or other significant cardiac pathology

- The competency proformas used to review and mark these cases are available at the BSE web address previously mentioned: they detail the echocardiographic features and measurements that your examiner will be looking for
- The examiners recognize there may be minor elements missing from the imaging data set where cases are performed in critical care areas. However, no key contextual or technical information should be missing entirely: these cases are highly selected and therefore should reflect your best practice.

Tips for successful ACCE accreditation

- Identify a willing supervisor who has the time, and skills to train you properly through to the end of the process: this is a big investment for your trainer, but fully training an intensive care clinician in

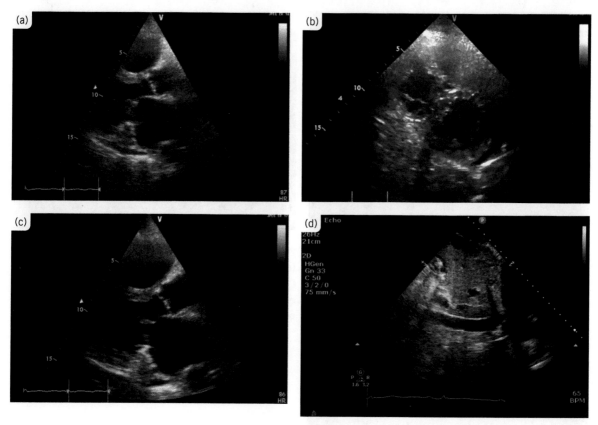

Figure 1.5 **(a) [Video 1.9], (b) [Video 1.10], (c) [Video 1.11], and (d) [Video 1.12] Gross hypovolaemia.**
🔘 *These videos are available to watch in the online video appendix.*
© Oxford University Hospitals NHS Foundation Trust 2016, with permission.

echocardiography will reduce the number of referrals into a hardworking outpatient echo department.

- It is recommended that at least 75 studies are performed in the outpatient setting: we would recommend cementing your imaging skills in the outpatient setting before attempting to image critically ill patients.

- Be clear with the critical care team that you cannot use your skills clinically until you have completed a reasonable amount of training: 100 cases is a good marker. From approximately this stage of your training, you should continue to perform some studies in outpatients, but the majority should be performed in patients requiring review or admission by critical care services.

- Tell your trainer early if you are not progressing: bear in mind that learning to

echo well is very similar to learning a musical instrument and requires frequent, regular practice. There are often small issues with technique that prevent you from progressing that can be corrected by your trainer.

- Learn to control your 'echo-hand' well before you try and use your other hand to optimize and measure at the same time. Holding a steady image is key to making correct observations.

- Do not expect to include every case you perform in your logbook. The logbook is a collection of selected cases that demonstrate a solid knowledge and experience base.

- Begin practising for, reviewing and re-attempting your demonstration cases early: it takes several months to find the right cases to submit for your five demonstration cases. Submitting five good cases

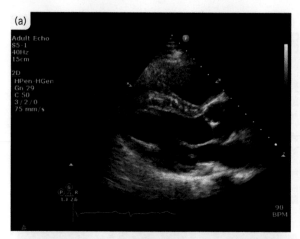

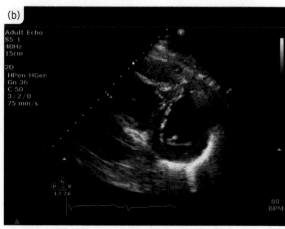

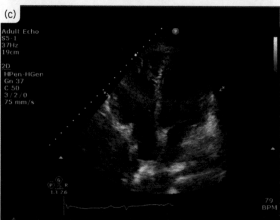

Figure 1.6 (a) [Video 1.13], (b) [Video 1.14], and (c) [Video 1.15] Acute right heart dysfunction.

These videos are available to watch in the online video appendix.

© Oxford University Hospitals NHS Foundation Trust 2016, with permission.

usually takes about ten attempts. Do not leave this to the last minute.

Echo for prognostication in critical illness

When we echo critically unwell patients, we must be mindful that we are looking at their cardiac anatomy and physiology as a snapshot during their illness, and not in a steady state.

Examples of where this is important are:

- Labelling patients with a high left ventricular end-diastolic pressure (LVEDP) as having diastolic dysfunction when their diastology is normal outside the context of their illness
- Labelling patients with a septic left ventricle (LV) as having systolic dysfunction

- Assessing mitral regurgitation (MR) grade when on noradrenaline.

Many echocardiographic features will return to baseline when the patient recovers from their critical illness; therefore, it is part of the critical care echocardiographer's role to recognize when a patient needs a repeat outpatient echo to clarify their true baseline cardiac structure and function and prevent misguiding future clinical assessment. This case study from our clinical practice illustrates this point.

CASE STUDY

The importance of re-assessing cardiac function following the resolution of critical illness

A 20-year-old lady with severe malnutrition was admitted to the critical care unit with a broad complex tachycardia and a very low systolic blood pressure. On examination, she was found to be cachexic, with peripheral oedema and a rash on the extensor aspect of her legs. She was cold peripherally to the knees and elbows and had a low-volume pulse.

A member of the critical care echo team was asked to perform an echocardiogram to help identify the cause of her cardiac instability. The key echo findings were:

- Evidence of left ventricular wall thinning and left ventricular dilatation
- Ejection fraction (EF) of 30%
- Estimated LVEDP of 20 mmHg using tissue Doppler and transmitral Doppler assessment of the E and E′ waves
- Diastolic dominance in pulmonary venous inflow trace
- Circumferential small-volume pericardial effusion.

These images are shown in Figures 1.7 (a) to (c) 🎥 and (d) to (f).

The echo was reported in the clinical context as demonstrating severe cardiomyopathy due to vitamin, trace element, protein, and calorie deficiency, with evidence of reduced left ventricular relaxation and raised LVEDP.

Over the next six weeks, she was managed with controlled refeeding, angiotensin-converting enzyme (ACE) inhibition, and negative fluid balance with serial echo monitoring to guide fluid management and re-assess left ventricular relaxation and LVEDP.

Follow-up echo at 12 weeks demonstrated normal ventricular thickness and shape, an EF of 45%, and partial normalization of diastolic function. She was followed up at six months and her echo was reported as normal.

Service models and quality indicators for satellite critical care echocardiography services

Critical care echocardiography is rapidly developing with a specific patient care remit and an immediate and measurable impact on patient care. It has therefore become vital that we can evidence the quality of what we do and that a central governing body provides guidance on quality standards.

Cardiology departments house echo services that are governed by the Departmental Accreditation Committee of the BSE. As yet, the BSE has not issued nationally agreed guidelines for departmental accreditation of critical care echo services, but it is likely to do so shortly.

The essential components of any service are structure, processes, and outcomes.

Structure

Staffing: identification of a Clinical Lead (CL) for the service and a link Consultant Cardiologist are the vital initial steps. Without adequate time and finance allocation for the Clinical Lead, the service cannot develop or be regulated. The Clinical Lead can be identified before they have achieved their final level of echo training; service development can run concurrently with personnel training. Formalization of their role will also help them to achieve their training aims through their personal development plan at appraisal.

Facilities: over time, the whole critical care team will become familiar with the process of critical care echo and the requirements for patient positioning prior to each study.

Equipment: capital investment into adequate echo equipment and storage licences is a vital primary step.

Processes

Requesting: this is one of the most difficult parts of the process to standardize. There are many potential ways to request an in-house critical care echo. The process chosen should fit into local practice and capture all requests.

Interpretation/reporting/documentation: all studies must be documented in the notes or electronic patient chart and re-interpreted for non-echocardiographers as a basic minimum. There should be a mechanism in place for senior review where the echocardiographer does not know how to report the echo findings in the patient context.

Outcomes

Monitoring: critical care echocardiography contrasts with outpatient departmental echocardiography in that the impact on patients is both immediate and identifiable. This should be monitored by the Clinical Lead as a significant quality marker.

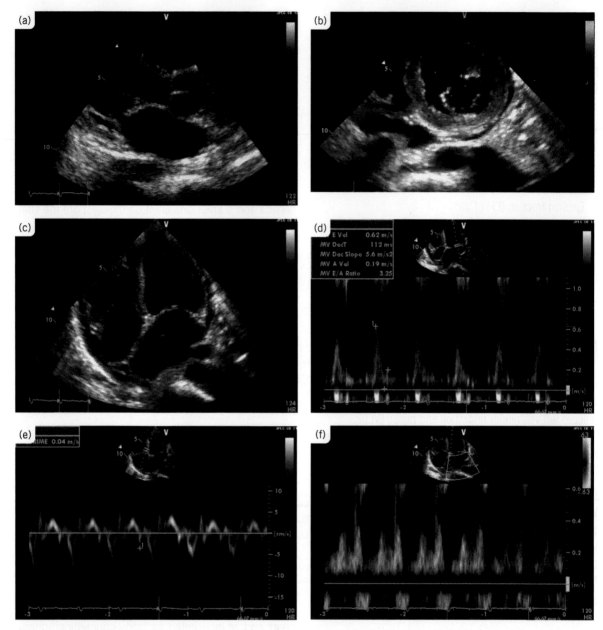

Figure 1.7 **(a)** [Video 1.16], **(b)** [Video 1.17], **(c)** [Video 1.18], and **(d)** to **(f)** **Parasternal long and short axis, apical four-chamber views, and interrogation of diastolic function to calculate the left ventricular end-diastolic pressure.**

⬤ *These videos are available to watch in the online video appendix.*

© Oxford University Hospitals NHS Foundation Trust 2016, with permission.

Service start-up

If you are planning to introduce a full critical care echo service into your department, considering each of these categories will ensure you set the service up to both perform and evidence a high-quality service from the outset.

Table 1.2 gives suggested standards for critical care echo services and highlights the strong links between training and service quality. We have given two categories of service provision to show how a unit may progress from predominantly FICE level scanning to performing full echo studies in most patients.

Table 1.2 Suggested quality indicators for in-house critical care echo services

Parameter	FICE accreditation teaching unit	BSE accreditation teaching unit
Structure		
Staffing	Appointed BSE-accredited CL	Appointed BSE-accredited CL with adequate PA allocation for service workload
	All echo team members: • Are identified • Are qualified (various levels) • Work within their qualification level • Take part in re-accreditation, including the CL	All echo team members: • Are identified • Are qualified (various levels) • Work within their qualification level • Take part in re-accreditation, including the CL • Attend regular quality review meetings
Facilities	Written standards are established and disseminated to the echo team defining: • Safe practice of bedside echo with multi-organ support • Optimization of patient positioning • Appropriate liaison with nursing team/duty medical team/patients/families Standards are role-modelled and maintained by the CL	Written standards are established and disseminated to the echo team defining: • Safe practice of bedside echo with multi-organ support • Optimization of patient positioning • Appropriate liaison with nursing team/duty medical team/patients/families Standards are role-modelled and maintained by the CL
Equipment	Portable equipment is: • <7 years old • equipped with relevant software storage packages • regularly serviced	Portable equipment is: • <7 years old • equipped with relevant software storage packages • regularly serviced
	Images are stored.	Images are stored on the central echo storage system There is a service line agreement in place for access to the central cardiology department storage facility to facilitate audit and expert review
	Reporting facilities will vary from unit to unit	Reporting and reviewing stations are accessible to all echo team members in critical care areas
Processes		
Requesting	All echo operators know the indications for a FICE echo and work within those guidelines	There is an agreed and disseminated list of indications for echo studies in the critically ill with agreed categories for: • Immediate • Urgent • Elective studies
	Studies are performed in a timely manner Time between referral and completion of a study could be audited	There are agreed time parameters for the provision of: • Immediate (30–60 min) • Urgent (2–4 hours) • Elective studies (within 48 hours) Documentation of referral time and study times in the notes allows auditing

Continued

13

Table 1.2 *Continued*

Parameter	FICE accreditation teaching unit	BSE accreditation teaching unit
	The CL ensures that FICE scans are repeated by a more skilled operator to achieve a BSE minimum data set where indicated	>75% of elective studies achieve the BSE minimum data set FICE scans are repeated, where indicated, to achieve a minimum data set
		The CL formulates, updates, and disseminates protocols for specific critical care indications as they become available
Interpretation reporting documentation	A written report is entered into the notes for every FICE study undertaken. The study should be labelled 'FICE scan'	A written report is entered into the patient's notes or electronic patient record for all studies and includes: • Time of referral • Time of study • Type of study: 'FICE scan' or 'ACCE' • Clinical question and • Describes all relevant parts of the heart • Provides an answer to the clinical question interpreted for the non-echocardiographer in the clinical context
	There is a nominated link cardiologist.	There is a nominated link cardiologist with whom the CL and other team members regularly liaise The critical care echo team attend and contribute to cardiology departmental echo review meetings
	There is access to a more advanced study within a clinically appropriate time frame	The CL establishes and disseminates a written protocol for the escalation of clinical queries
Service maintenance	The CL disseminates written information on local policy for machine cleaning after use in: • Non-contaminated • Contaminated areas. Machine cleaning is carried out after each study	The CL disseminates written information on local policy for machine cleaning after use in: • Non-contaminated • Contaminated areas Machine cleaning is carried out after each study
Outcomes		
Study outcomes	The CL fully audits the echo service two-yearly and takes action to improve the service in identified weak areas These audits and actions are documented	The CL fully audits the echo service two-yearly and takes action to improve the service in identified weak areas These audits and actions are documented

CL, Clinical Lead.

Reproduced with permission from TC Thomas and CL Colebourn, 'Measuring and monitoring quality in satellite echo services within critical care: an exploration of best practice', *Echo Research and Practice*, 2, 2, pp. 57–64, Copyright © 2015 The Authors.

Training processes and evaluation

One of the most important functions of a critical care echo service is to train both future clinical leads in critical care echo and clinicians using the FICE protocol.

A safe and high-quality in-house critical care echo service is the strongest structure within which to train, providing a standardized method of senior review and immediate access to an expert opinion where the answer to a clinical question is unclear.

Our training experience over the past nine years has helped us to identify some important tips for successfully housing a training system within a service structure:

1. Group FICE trainees together to a set time each week where their cases can be reviewed. They learn from each other and this prevents the trainers from receiving ad hoc requests throughout the working week for review of a single echo study; this becomes very time-inefficient

2. Consultants or senior trainees who have decided to pursue ACCE will not achieve accreditation within two years without dedicated identified scanning time with a trainer who is allocated to them for that period. We recommend a minimum of one session per week over a two year period for a consultant undertaking ACCE accreditation and a regular half or whole-day of training for a senior trainee undertaking the same process

3. In the same way that the quality of an echo service needs careful monitoring, so too does the quality of educational process. Having a mechanism in place for regular review of trainee echocardiographers' progress is vital to re-initiate positive progress where it is stalling.

Picking up a new detailed practical skill such as echocardiography never progresses in a linear motion and a two-way process of evaluation should be in place to prevent derailment. This is most applicable to those undertaking advanced training.

If you want to set up a satellite critical care echo service and need help and advice, please contact us at the Oxford Critical Care Fellowship and we will be happy to help (Claire.colebourn@ouh.nhs.uk).

Further reading

Alam SR, Docherty A, Mackle I, Gillies MA. The introduction of intensive care-led echocardiography into a tertiary care unit. *JICS* 2013; **14**: 15–19.

British Society of Echocardiography. *A minimum dataset for a standard transthoracic echocardiogram.* http://bsecho. azurewebsites.net/media/71250/tte_ds_sept_2012.pdf.

Bruemmer-Smith S, Colebourn C, Fletcher N; The Joint British Society of Echocardiography and Intensive Care Society Committee for Critical Care Echocardiography and Committee for Focused Intensive Care Echocardiography. Accreditation for critical care echocardiography. *JICS* 2012; **13**: 196–7.

Cecconi M, De Backer D, Antonelli M, *et al.* Concensus of circulatory shock and haemodynamic monitoring. Task force of the European Society of Intensive Care Medicine. Maurizio Cecconi, Daniel De Backer etal. *Intensive Care Med* 2014; **40**: 1795–815.

Colebourn CL, Barber V, Salmon JB, Young JD. The accuracy of diagnostic and haemodynamic data obtained by transthoracic echocardiography in critically ill adults: a systematic review. *JICS* 2008; **9**: 128–34.

Colebourn CL, Davies IKG, Becher H. Bridging the gap: training critical care clinician-echocardiographers through a collaborative curriculum. *JICS* 2010; **11**: 13–16.

Colebourn C, Jones L. Contemporary evaluation for medical ultrasound teachers. *Ultrasound* 2013; **21**: 57–63.

Thomas TC, Colebourn CL. Measuring and monitoring quality in satellite echo services within critical care: an exploration of best practice. *Echo Res Pract* June 2015; **2**: 57–64.

2

The left ventricle in critical illness

Assessing the circulatory system in critical illness

Relationship between systolic performance, ejection fraction, and clinical context.

The echocardiographic term often used to describe systolic function is ejection fraction (EF).

In the strictest sense, however, EF should be viewed as a load-**dependent** measure of left ventricular work determined by a combination of:

1. Myocyte work determined by underlying and current power capacity
2. Fluid balance
3. Cardiovascular drugs
4. Overall clinical state
5. Heart rate and rhythm.

In clinical practice, the predominant planes of contraction used to determine left ventricular contractility are radial thickening and longitudinal shortening, as shown in Figure 2.1.

Echocardiography allows the clinician to make an integrated assessment of left ventricular performance in a short time frame, with particular reference to:

1. Contractility and interaction of both the left and right ventricles
2. Causes of chronic or acute contractile failure—both global and regional
3. Other pathologies that significantly alter the cardiac output generated by cardiac work done, for example valve pathology and pericardial fluid.

Load-**independent** measures of systolic performance are available, for example strain rate imaging, but these techniques are not yet reliably performed at the bedside in a time frame relevant to the critically ill patient.

Practice point

Contraction of the left ventricle (LV) is a complex multidimensional process. Hence, there are significant risks in estimating or measuring myocardial work from a single measure. Best practice should triangulate qualitative and quantitative estimates and measures of ventricular work and place that workload within the clinical context.

Measuring and estimating ejection fraction

EF describes the ratio of the total end-diastolic volume that is ejected by the end of systole. Measurements at the end of diastole and systole are therefore required to make these assessments. Measurements should be timed to the cardiac cycle, using the electrocardiogram (ECG) trace wherever possible.

The quantitative measures of left ventricular performance given in 'Quantitative measures of ejection fraction' below should be triangulated to the echocardiographer's qualitative assessment of ventricular function which should be practised enough to gauge whether a ventricle has near-normal, normal, mild, moderate, or severely subnormal performance.

When routinely practised, qualitative assessment has been shown to correlate well with measured variables, although interobserver variation must be taken into account.

(a)

(b)

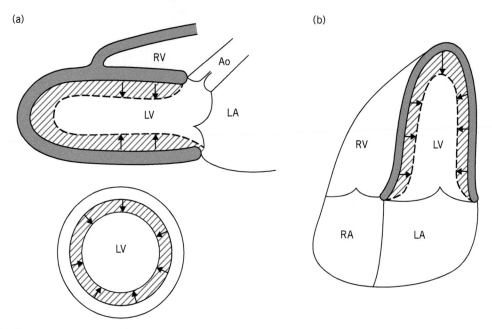

Figure 2.1 **Diagram of the left ventricle demonstrating the direction of myocardial thickening during systole in the parasternal long and short, and apical windows.**

Practice point

Best practice should include:

- Quantitative assessment to provide a reproducible and repeatable parameter and
- Qualitative assessment to guard against measurement or numerical errors producing an EF that does not reflect what the echocardiographer is seeing.

Quantitative measures of ejection fraction

Single plane measurements

Linear measurements

Fractional shortening
Assessment of the diameter of the LV during systole and diastole can be used to generate an estimate of the EF. The traditional approach uses the M-mode in the parasternal long-axis (PLAX) view, with the cursor placed perpendicular to the walls just **below** the tips of the mitral valve leaflets in systole. Measurement of the diameter of the LV cavity during systole and diastole produces a simple assessment of left ventricular performance. This measure is referred to as fractional

shortening (FS). EF can then be calculated from FS using the following formula, with values obtained as shown in Figure 2.2.

$$[(LVIDd - LVIDs)/LVIDd] \times 100 = FS\%$$

The use of M-mode imaging provides superior temporal resolution that allows for precise measurements but relies upon a correctly aligned calliper. The calliper should be

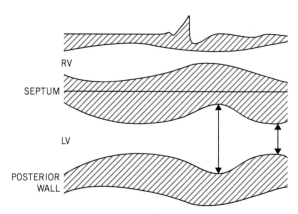

Figure 2.2 **Diagram of M-mode assessment of the left ventricle to generate an estimate of fractional shortening.**

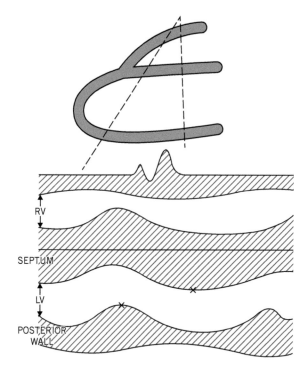

Figure 2.3 Diagram of M-mode left ventricular assessment, demonstrating the impact of using an off-axis cut to generate fractional shortening values.

placed at 90 degrees to the axis of the ventricular walls to avoid diagonal cuts, as shown in Figure 2.3. When using M-mode, measurements must be made using the leading edge to leading edge technique to ensure that consistent, reproducible measurements are produced. When the LV is best imaged in the PLAX view off axis, two-dimensional (2D) imaging and point-to-point measurements should be used in preference.

Practice point

When using M-mode to perform linear measurements, accepted practice is the use of leading edge measurements. This technique starts measuring at the first line generated by a structure and is followed throughout, thereby creating uniform, reproducible, and consistent values.

MAPSE

Mitral annular plane systolic excursion (MAPSE) is an alternative single-view, linear left ventricular performance measure that examines the descent of the lateral mitral annulus using the apical four-chamber view. MAPSE can be used to quantify the longitudinal function of the LV. The measure is not useful alone since it looks solely at the basal longitudinal function of the LV and is therefore misleading in the presence of both regional wall motion abnormalities and radial dysfunction. An M-mode calliper is placed across the lateral annulus of the LV using the apical four-chamber view and a spectral M-mode trace is displayed on the screen, similar to the technique used in generating a tricuspid annular plane systolic excursion (TAPSE). The maximal systolic excursion is measured and displayed in milimetres.

Practice point

MAPSE can be a useful representation of left ventricular function in the absence of regional wall motion abnormalities. The normal range is 12 ± 2 mm.

Area measurements

Fractional area change

Fractional area change (FAC) is an alternative approach to a single-view estimate of the EF that examines end-systolic and end-diastolic areas of the LV at the mid-papillary level in the parasternal short-axis view. As shown in Figure 2.4, the FAC is calculated by tracing the end-diastolic and end-systolic areas and is calculated using the following equation:

$$(\text{End-diastolic area}) - (\text{End-systolic area}) \ / \ (\text{End-diastolic area}) \times 100\%$$

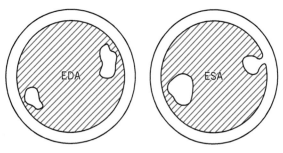

Figure 2.4 Diagram of the left ventricle at the mid-papillary level in the parasternal short axis view. The cross-sectional area of the left ventricle is estimated at end-diastole and end-systole. This generates a useful estimate of the fractional area change. EDA, end-diastolic area; ESA, end-systolic area.

Since the majority of left ventricular performance is radial, estimates of the FAC have been shown to correlate well with volumetric methods of left ventricular assessment. Short-axis visualization of the LV is frequently feasible in critically ill patients, using either the parasternal or modified subcostal short-axis views. Care must be taken when choosing the level at which FAC measurement is performed. The apex and basal segments must be avoided since the apex obliterates completely during systole due to its predominantly circumferential wringing motion, and the basal segments remain relatively fixed due to their cartilaginous connections.

Practice point

To allow for accurate, reproducible FAC measurements, the mid-papillary level offers an easily identifiable anatomical landmark that functionally reflects the LV in the absence of significant regional wall motion abnormalities.

Doppler measurements of ejection fraction

Estimating stroke volume and cardiac output

Doppler can be used to estimate the systolic performance of the LV by providing a measurement of the stroke volume (SV) calculated from the transvalvular velocity and the valve area. SV can be measured across any valve, assuming no shunt or significant regurgitation is present, but is most often measured at the aortic valve since the aortic outflow tract is circular and the diameter cleanly measured in the PLAX view.

SV is multiplied by heart rate to provide a volume estimate of cardiac output that **must** be interpreted in the context of quantitative and qualitative assessment of the LV. The main source of error in this measurement is the left ventricular outflow tract (LVOT) diameter, which is squared to estimate the area of the valve. The process of estimating SV is shown in Figure 2.5 with the accompanying formula.

Practice point

Transaortic assessment of SV and cardiac output is a commonly used, repeatable, and useful measure of EF in the critical care setting.

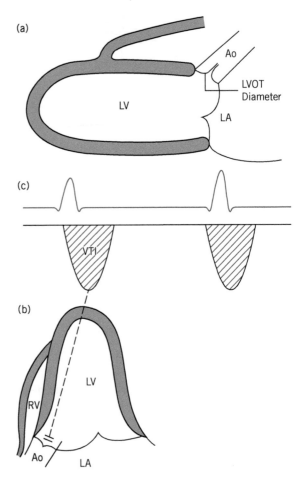

Figure 2.5 Diagram of stroke volume measurement using transthoracic echocardiography. The diameter of the LVOT is measured with the aortic valve open, as shown in diagram (a). A pulsed-wave Doppler calliper is placed at the corresponding position in the apical five-chamber view, as shown in diagram (b) to produce a spectral trace, as shown in diagram (c). Measurement of the velocity time integral (VTI) of this trace is integrated with the diameter of the LVOT to generate an estimate of stroke volume. Stroke volume = π (LVOT diameter / 2)^2 × LVOT VTI (a) PLAX. Position to measure the LVOT with the valve open in ventricular systole. (b) Apical five-chamber. Pulsed-wave calliper position at the same level as the LVOT measurement in PLAX. (c) Pulsed-wave spectral trace with VTI tracing to generate stroke volume measurement.

Pressure/time gradient

The angle of a velocity gradient can be used to derive a measure of work or power. In clinical practice, an MR jet can provide us with a Doppler trace on which this can be done, giving us an inverse reflection of the left ventricular work. By measuring the time taken for the velocity to increase from 1 m/s to 3 m/s along a continuous-wave Doppler trace, we can determine the change in pressure over time. This technique is demonstrated in Figure 2.6.

Despite being relatively load-independent, the requirement for at least moderate MR, the technical difficulties in obtaining an accurate Doppler envelope, and the assumption of negligible left atrial pressure limit the clinical usefulness of this method.

Tissue Doppler imaging

Tissue Doppler imaging (TDi) operates in exactly the same way as the spectral Doppler measurements of blood cell velocities we are used to seeing. To measure blood cell velocities, the probe filters out low velocities and accentuates the high-velocity, low-amplitude movements of the red blood cells as they pass through the circulation. When switched to the TDi mode, the filters are reversed and the probe selects out and displays low-velocity, high-amplitude signals from the muscular walls of the heart.

Tissue Doppler assessment of the LV can therefore generate information about systolic function. A typical TDi trace obtained from the base of the LV via the apical window is shown in Figure 2.7. TDi demonstrates the maximum velocity of the **specific region** of the myocardium being imaged and therefore cannot be used as a global cardiac assessment without multiple measurements being taken.

Practice point

Although additive, TDi does not provide comprehensive information on left ventricular function and EF alone. Normal ranges for basal lateral and medial walls vary according to age; however, values <6 cm/s for septal and 8 cm/s for lateral walls usually represent abnormally low systolic function.

Tei index

By integrating transmitral pulsed-wave Doppler measurements with transaortic flow times, the Tei index can be calculated. Devised by Tei Chuwa in 1995 as an index of myocardial performance, both systolic and diastolic performance are integrated to provide an overall picture of left ventricular function.

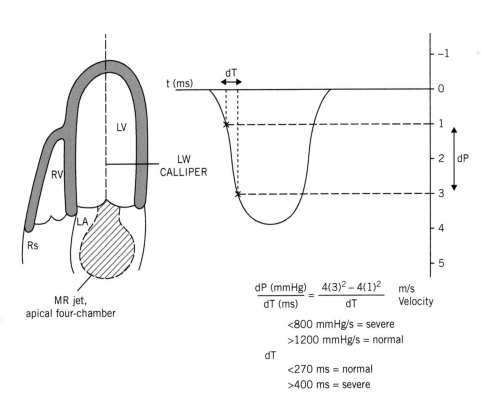

$$\frac{dP \ (mmHg)}{dT \ (ms)} = \frac{4(3)^2 - 4(1)^2}{dT} \quad \begin{array}{l} m/s \\ Velocity \end{array}$$

<800 mmHg/s = severe
>1200 mmHg/s = normal

dT
<270 ms = normal
>400 ms = severe

Figure 2.6 Diagram demonstrating the technique used to perform the dP/dT technique. Using the apical four-chamber view, a continuous-wave calliper is placed through the tips of the mitral valve leaflets and the jet of mitral regurgitation. The spectral trace is optimized to display a maximal velocity of at least 4 m/s. The time taken for the velocity to increase from 1 m/s to 3 m/s allows calculation of the dP/dT ratio.

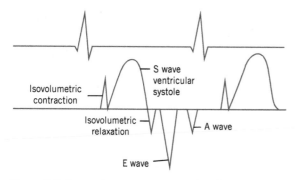

Figure 2.7 Spectral trace generated using tissue Doppler settings to demonstrate movement of the LV during the normal cardiac cycle. The peak velocity of the S wave is used as a marker of systolic performance.

A transmitral Doppler signal is obtained at the tips of the mitral valve leaflets in the apical four-chamber view to measure the duration of transmitral flow. A similar measurement is made at the base of the LVOT below the aortic valve leaflets to measure the ejection time. By comparing the ratio of these two time intervals, an index is generated that has been shown to be relatively preload-independent and of useful prognostic value in cardiology cohorts. The practical use of this conglomerate measure of left ventricular systolic and diastolic function is yet to be determined in critically ill patients. Figure 2.8 demonstrates the measurement of the Tei index and associated normal ranges.

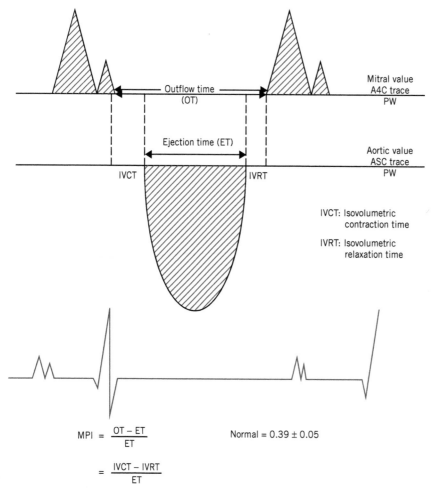

Figure 2.8 Diagram demonstrating how to perform the Tei index when estimating myocardial performance.

Biplane measurements

Using more than one measurement plane should improve the accuracy with which we can estimate the EF. An estimate of the ejected volume of blood from the LV can be calculated using the modified hemisphere cylinder formula, also known as the bullet formula. The same technique can be used at end-systole to generate an EF.

$$\left[\begin{array}{c} 5 \times \text{LV CSA (mid-papillary PSAX)} \\ \times \text{length (A4C, end-diastole)} \end{array} \right] / 6$$

Simpson's biplane method

Use of the formula requires measurement of the left ventricular endocardial border, followed by measurement of the length of the LV from the base to the apex. The Simpson's biplane method employs this technique in two separate planes, more accurately reflecting the impact of individual regional wall motion abnormalities on the overall EF in a proportionate way.

The Simpson's biplane method uses the apical four- and two-chamber views. Tracings of the endocardium of the LV at end-systole and end-diastole are performed in both views, and a longitudinal measurement of the LV is added. The subsequent three-dimensional (3D) model created by the imaging software is divided into 20 stacked discs that represent the ascending regional volumes at each level of the LV. These individual volumes are collated to produce an accurate estimate of EF, as shown in Figure 2.9.

> ### Practice point
>
> Clear endocardial definition is required for accurate estimation of EF using this method since area measurement errors are exaggerated to the power of three by the hemisphere formula. The use of contrast can significantly improve the definition of the left ventricular endocardium in patients with suboptimal windows, and development of automated techniques (automated border detection, speckle tracking) may improve both the accuracy and reproducibility of this technique in the future.

A summary of the categorization and practical use of these assessments of left ventricular function are given in Table 2.1. The practical integration of these measurement techniques is demonstrated in the following case study.

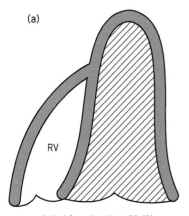

(a)

Apical four-chamber with LV
traced at end-diastole

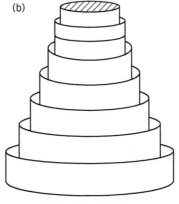

(b)

Series of stacked discs
used to represent chamber
volume for biplane estimation

Figure 2.9 Diagram of the biplane process and stacked discs. (a): apical four-chamber with the left ventricle traced at end-diastole. (b): series of stacked discs used to represent the chamber volume for biplane estimation.

Table 2.1 A summary of the methods available at the bedside for assessing left ventricular performance using transthoracic echocardiography. The techniques are grouped according to the number of planes required to generate the values being used, along with relevant pitfalls and merits

Technique category	Technique principle	Technique	Imaging method	Useful when/to	Use should be avoided when
Single plane	Linear	FS	PLAX comparison of basal LV in systole/diastole	Screening assessment of global function	RWMA present Poor windows
		MAPSE	Apical four-chamber, M-mode at lateral and medial annulus	Assess longitudinal systolic function	RWMA
	Area	FAC	Short axis view of LV at mid-papillary level	Cornerstone of left ventricular assessment	Basal/apical RWMA
	Doppler	Cardiac output measurement	Pulsed wave Doppler appropriately placed	Measurement of cardiac output	Associated valvular pathology
		TDi	S-wave peak velocity	Combined with other techniques Suboptimal windows	RWMA
		Tei index	Apical four-chamber	Most load-independent measure of left ventricular contractility	Technical difficulty and accuracy in identifying isovolaemic stages
		dP/dT	Continuous wave Doppler through MR trace	At least moderate MR. Good screening for normal and severe left ventricular impairment Relatively independent of loading conditions	No/mild MR
Biplane	Area	Area length equation	Area measurement of LV in systole and diastole, combined with length measurement from A4C	Screening of global function	Non-geometric LV (i.e. old, hypertensive) RWMA Structural abnormality, i.e. left ventricular aneurysm
	Volume	Simpson's biplane method	Apical four- and two-chamber	Good endocardial definition	Poor windows
3D	Volume	Multiplanar Simpson's method	Apical window	Good endocardial definition Machine with 3D capability	Poor windows/definition

3D, three-dimensional; MR, mitral regurgitation; RWMA, regional wall motion abnormalities.

CASE STUDY

Fixing broken hearts—stress cardiomyopathy, diagnosis, and evolution of reversible cardiomyopathy

A 56-year-old female was admitted via the emergency department with sudden-onset collapse precipitated by severe headache. Computed tomography (CT) scanning confirmed the presence of a subarachnoid haemorrhage, and the patient was transferred to the intensive care department to facilitate supportive care. On admission, she was tachycardic and hypertensive. An ECG demonstrated sinus rhythm with non-specific ST- and T-wave changes, and high-sensitivity troponin was mildly elevated. Bedside echocardiography revealed a borderline hyperdynamic heart, but no other significant abnormalities (Figure 2.10 ▣).

Over the next 24 hours, the patient developed signs and symptoms consistent with shock. She was cool peripherally with prolonged capillary refill, and arterial blood gas analysis revealed an elevated lactate level. She was aggressively fluid-loaded to facilitate clearance of her lactate. Following initial improvements in lactate values and urine output, subsequent development of

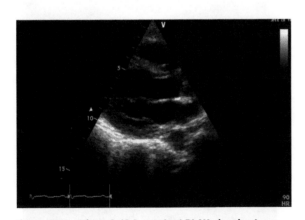

Figure 2.10 [Video 2.1] A standard PLAX view is shown here, with all segments visualized contracting normally. The valve structure and function is within normal limits and the ejection fraction is at the upper limit of normal.

▣ *This video is available to watch in the online video appendix.*

© Oxford University Hospitals NHS Foundation Trust 2016, with permission.

hypotension resulted in commencement of an infusion of noradrenaline which was steadily rising by day 2. Repeat troponin values were markedly elevated; however, the ECG remained unremarkable.

An urgent TTE was requested to assess left ventricular function and assist in prioritizing clinical management.

Figures 2.11 to 2.15 ▣ were taken 24 hours following admission to critical care, and the striking abnormality is the fall in systolic performance of the LV. The regions shown in the long axis and short axis are globally impaired, except the basal regions which remain hyperdynamic. There has been a subsequent fall in the overall EF. Whilst the apex is significantly impaired, it does not demonstrate the classical apical ballooning seen in Takotsubo.

After discussion with cardiology, a screening coronary angiogram was performed, which demonstrated no obstructing lesion within the coronary circulation, and an intra-aortic balloon pump was inserted. Significant improvements in blood pressure and cardiac output values followed the initiation of an infusion of dobutamine at 15 micrograms/kg/min. Over the next 7 days, the inotropic support was weaned successfully, and a repeat echocardiogram revealed normal left ventricular function before discharge 1 week later.

When Figures 2.16 to 2.19 ▣ are compared with the previous images, the overall left ventricular contractility has significantly improved, and this is predominantly due to improvements in mid-papillary and apical contractility. The overall EF is restored to normal values, and the appearance of the previously affected regions of the myocardium has also normalized, in keeping with the diagnosis of reversible stress cardiomyopathy.

Understanding circulation in sepsis

Septic shock is a common indication for management in a critical care area. Sepsis is defined in clinical practice as a systemic inflammatory process, triggered by infection, with subsequent changes in the circulation and organ function.

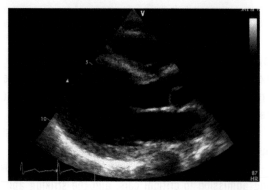

Figure 2.11 [Video 2.2] A PLAX showing severely impaired left ventricular systolic impairment, apart from the basal regions, which still thicken relatively well.

🎥 *This video is available to watch in the online video appendix.*

© Oxford University Hospitals NHS Foundation Trust 2016, with permission.

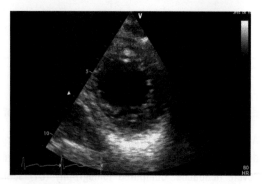

Figure 2.12 [Video 2.3] A parasternal short axis apical view, revealing severely impaired systolic function.
Instead of completely obliterating the ventricular cavity during systole, a significant end-systolic area remains, representing severe systolic impairment. Whilst the apical function is impaired, it does not demonstrate the classical dilation described in Takutsubo's cardiomyopathy.

🎥 *This video is available to watch in the online video appendix.*

© Oxford University Hospitals NHS Foundation Trust 2016, with permission.

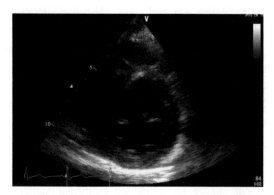

Figure 2.13 [Video 2.4] Further impairment of the left ventricular systolic function with globally reduced systolic work throughout the mid-papillary level of the left ventricle.

🎥 *This video is available to watch in the online video appendix.*

© Oxford University Hospitals NHS Foundation Trust 2016, with permission.

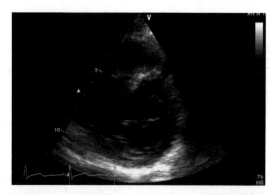

Figure 2.14 [Video 2.5] Basal function remains relatively preserved when assessed using the parasternal short axis basal view, in keeping with the regionality demonstrated in the PLAX views.

🎥 *This video is available to watch in the online video appendix.*

© Oxford University Hospitals NHS Foundation Trust 2016, with permission.

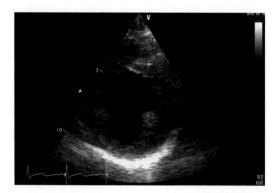

Figure 2.15 [Video 2.6] This video further demonstrates the degree of systolic impairment at the mid-papillary level of the parasternal short axis, showing global left ventricular impairment.

🎥 *This video is available to watch in the online video appendix.*

© Oxford University Hospitals NHS Foundation Trust 2016, with permission.

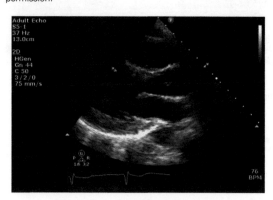

Figure 2.16 [Video 2.7] A repeat PLAX performed 1 week after developing left ventricular impairment. The PLAX shows a significant improvement in global systolic work, compared with Video 2.2.

🎥 *This video is available to watch in the online video appendix.*

© Oxford University Hospitals NHS Foundation Trust 2016, with permission.

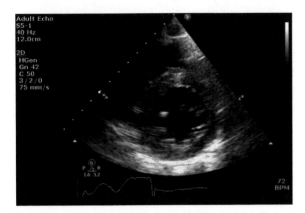

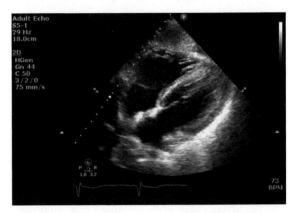

Figure 2.17 [Video 2.8] This video demonstrates relatively normal radial thickening at the papillary muscle level using the parasternal short axis.

🎥 *This video is available to watch in the online video appendix.*
© Oxford University Hospitals NHS Foundation Trust 2016, with permission.

Figure 2.19 [Video 2.10] A subcostal long axis further confirms the return of overall left ventricular systolic function to normal ranges.

🎥 *This video is available to watch in the online video appendix.*
© Oxford University Hospitals NHS Foundation Trust 2016, with permission.

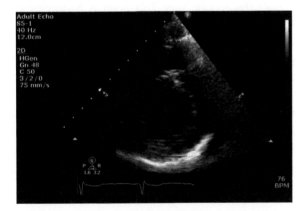

Figure 2.18 [Video 2.9] Apical function is restored to normal levels at the same stage, as shown in Video 2.9. The global apical systolic function has significantly improved when compared to Video 2.3.

🎥 *This video is available to watch in the online video appendix.*
© Oxford University Hospitals NHS Foundation Trust 2016, with permission.

Often the dominant clinical findings are profound arterial vasodilation and a high cardiac output state. Therapeutic strategies are therefore focused on optimizing volume status and restoring systemic arterial tone, in an attempt to restore organ perfusion pressure.

The phenomenon of left ventricular impairment as a direct result of the septic process has been known about and studied for over 50 years. Early observational studies of patients with septic shock described two distinct phases or patterns of shock:

- Sepsis in association with warm peripheries: vasodilatory shock
- Sepsis in association with cold peripheries: low cardiac output state.

The latter was regarded as carrying a significantly higher mortality rate.

Further evidence of a significant incidence of low cardiac output state amongst patients with sepsis has recently emerged from more sophisticated studies, which have demonstrated impaired cardiac contractility in the setting of sepsis using a variety of techniques and at various stages of admission to critical care. Current estimates of the incidence of acute left ventricular impairment due to sepsis range from 20% to 70%, whilst right ventricular dysfunction is identified in up to 30% of cases. In addition, various studies have demonstrated elevations in biomarkers indicating cardiac damage, including troponin, creatine kinase (CK), and B-natriuretic peptide, due solely to the multi-organ process occurring during sepsis.

Pathological process of ventricular dysfunction in sepsis

Macroscopic changes to coronary artery flow do not appear central to the process of cardiac impairment during sepsis. This has been evidenced by normal angiograms and variable, but inconsistent, electrocardiographic changes at the time of presentation.

A hallmark of acute septic cardiomyopathy is its complete reversibility in survivors, suggesting a transient aetiology is responsible. Two of the most commonly postulated explanations for acute cardiac depression in sepsis are circulating inflammatory mediators with direct myocardial depressant effects and super-stimulation of intracardiac adrenoreceptors, resulting in acute tachyphylaxis and receptor downregulation. Adrenoreceptor tachyphylaxis is also seen in other pathological situations associated with massive adrenergic surge, such as subarachnoid haemorrhage, and can lead to transient regional wall motion abnormalities such as Takotsubo's cardiomyopathy.

During stress, cardiac muscle switches from predominantly fat metabolism at rest to metabolize and take up carbohydrate fuel sources. This occurs partly due to adrenoreceptor activation. Sepsis invokes a state of relative insulin resistance, and therefore, in combination, fuel switching and insulin resistance may contribute to reduced cardiac work at a given preload. Finally, left ventricular fatigue may occur as a result of prolonged, uncorrected vasodilation and uncoupling of high cardiac workload in combination with the above-mentioned temporal factors.

Although it was postulated in the 1970s that the cardiac response to sepsis reflected a state of hibernation and was associated with better patient outcomes, this has not been borne out in subsequent studies. Evidence of ventricular impairment in sepsis is a marker of disease severity and, although not found to be independently associated with a mortality effect, will contribute to changing prognosis, as every temporal component of critical illness does.

A changing algorithm for sepsis care

Many cardiac output monitors, such as the pulmonary artery catheter and peripheral continuous cardiac output monitors, can provide a single-point or continuous numerical description of cardiac output. The risk of using these values alone is that we cannot know the context of these individual values within a particular patient's Starling curve. Without additional information about the function of the ventricle and the right heart, we cannot interpret the values in the correct therapeutic way. This point is illustrated in Figure 2.20. Both show the point position of a cardiac output of 5.5 L, but in two different clinical circumstances. The management of each of these patients is very different.

Critical care echocardiography provides us with the tool we need to put our understanding of the impact of sepsis on the ventricle into practice. We are then in a position to assess the circulation more comprehensively in the septic patient, considering:

- The large vascular circulation: to guide fluid balance and requirements
- The small vascular circulation: to guide vasopressor requirements
- The left heart: to guide blood pressure targets balanced against the risk of super-vasconstriction to the heart, and identification of the failing ventricle
- The right heart: objective assessment of right ventricular systolic work in the context of septic shock, with or without mechanical ventilation.

This opinion is reflected in the recently published consensus guidelines on haemodynamic monitoring by

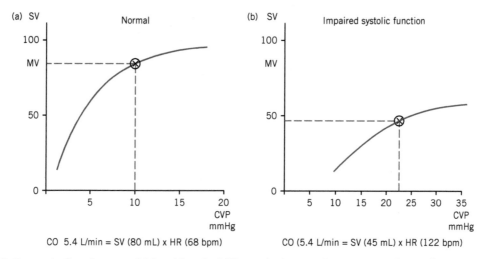

Figure 2.20 Demonstration of a normal (a) and impaired (b) ventricular systolic response to increasing preload.
Calculations of equivalent cardiac outputs demonstrate primary compensation occurs with an increased heart rate to try and maintain overall macroscopic flow.

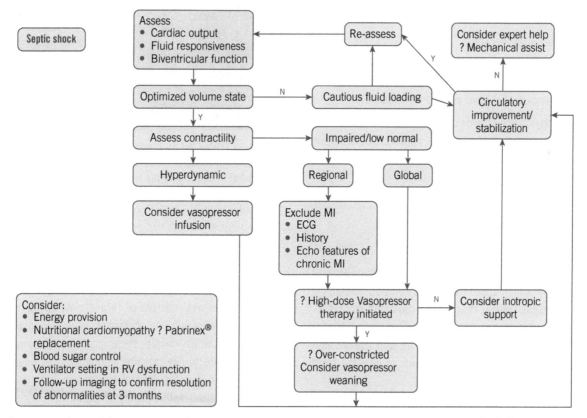

Figure 2.21 Systematic approach to the shocked septic patient, integrating echocardiographic assessment linked to therapeutic options.

the European Society of Intensive Care Medicine. The use of echocardiography is now suggested as the initial tool of choice when further haemodynamic assessment is needed. This represents a significant change in recommended clinical practice from the previous position of only using echocardiography when evidence of ventricular failure already existed.

Practice point

There is now recognition that systolic dysfunction is both more common than traditionally recognized and poorly identified by forms of circulatory assessment that provide only a numerical description of cardiac output and function.

Managing the septic ventricle

There is no single agent that can alleviate the dysfunction of a septic circulation. Figure 2.21 describes how we should consider each part of the circulation, as described earlier, to achieve an adequate circulation using:

- Titrated fluid therapy

- Vasopressors in vasodilatory shock: see Figure 8.3 in Chapter 8 for calculation of systemic vascular resistance (SVR) from echo-derived parameters

- Inotropy or other forms of ventricular support such as electrolytes and B vitamins where cardiac output is poor.

CASE STUDY

Impact of sepsis on the left ventricle

A 23-year-old previously fit and well female driver was involved in a high-speed road traffic collision, sustaining minor musculoskeletal injuries. Two days post-admission, following increasing abdominal pain, CT scanning demonstrated a bowel perforation, coinciding with the development of hypotension, tachycardia, and an elevated blood lactate level.

An emergency laparotomy was performed which confirmed a small bowel perforation and purulent peritonitis. Perioperatively, she was profoundly hypotensive, despite large-volume fluid resuscitation and multiple boluses of an

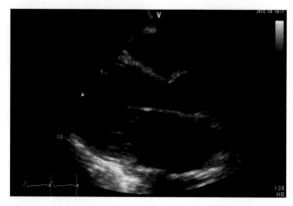

Figure 2.22 [Video 2.11] A severely impaired left ventricle which is non-dilated.

This video is available to watch in the online video appendix.
© Oxford University Hospitals NHS Foundation Trust 2016, with permission.

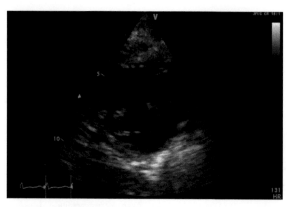

Figure 2.23 [Video 2.12] A mid-papillary short axis using the parasternal window, revealing significant impairment to the radial thickening of the left ventricle, with subsequent impact in left ventricular systolic work.

This video is available to watch in the online video appendix.
© Oxford University Hospitals NHS Foundation Trust 2016, with permission.

alpha agonist. Central venous access was secured, revealing a central venous pressure of 14 and a mixed venous oxygen saturation of 86%. An infusion of noradrenaline was commenced; however, despite these measures, the blood lactate continued to rise, coupled with ongoing deranged haemodynamics. A bolus dose of terlipressin 1 mg was administered, along with 200 mg of intravenous hydrocortisone, for presumed refractory septic shock. A lack of response to these measures prompted a damage control approach for the laparotomy to facilitate urgent transfer to

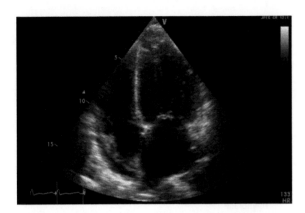

Figure 2.24 [Video 2.13] This demonstrates that this impairment extends down to the apex of the left ventricle. In an attempt to compensate for the degree of systolic impairment, the heart rate is elevated in order to maintain the cardiac output.

🔘 *This video is available to watch in the online video appendix.*
© Oxford University Hospitals NHS Foundation Trust 2016, with permission.

critical care. Bedside echocardiography was performed as the patient was admitted post-operatively to the intensive care unit (ICU). Transthoracic images from the parasternal long and short axis, and apical four-chamber are shown in Figures 2.22, 2.23, and 2.24 🔘. The right ventricle (RV) is seen to contract within normal limits and appears adequately filled, making hypovolaemia less likely as an explanation for the circulatory instability.

Following the echocardiogram, an infusion of dobutamine was commenced, whilst cautiously reducing the dose of the vasopressor guided by echocardiographic measures of cardiac output. Subsequent improvements in haemodyamics followed, as evidenced by improvements in organ function and falling blood lactate levels. The patient stabilized over the next 48 hours and returned to the operating theatre for closure of the laparotomy, before being extubated 4 days into ICU admission.

Important toxic drug effects on ventricular function

Pharmacological manipulation of cardiac performance is the intended outcome of a large number of drugs prescribed to manage or prevent cardiac arrhythmias or coronary disease. In relative or intended overdose, these drugs can cause circulatory collapse, which requires urgent and specific treatment. Rapid echocardiographic assessment provides the means for early recognition of the mechanism of circulatory collapse and then becomes a vital tool to guide restoration of the circulation.

Drugs causing idiosyncratic cardiac failure

Chemotherapy agents can cause idiosyncratic drug-induced heart failure by an unknown mechanism. Agents implicated include anthracyclines such as doxorubicin, cyclophosphamide, and taxanes such as paclitaxel, herceptin, and 5-fluorouracil. Idiosyncratic drug-induced heart failure due to chemotherapy agents can occur rapidly and at any stage of treatment. Selective cyclo-oxygenase 2 (COX-2) inhibitors have been shown to increase cardiovascular mortality when taken for sustained periods and are currently not licensed for administration in patients with cardiac disease.

New immunomodulating agents, such as interferon alpha, have been implicated in cases of acute reversible heart failure, whilst agents known to cause indirect heart failure due to rhythm disturbance, such as the tricyclic antidepressant amitryptiline, have been shown to have a direct negative inotropic effect as well. Anaesthetic agents can have direct negative inotropic effects and include volatile agents such as enflurane and intravenous agents such as barbiturates. Propofol, a lipid-soluble hypnotic/sedative drug commonly used in the management of the critically ill patient, is thought to produce hypotension predominantly via peripheral vasodilation; however, in excessive doses, it can precipitate an idiosyncratic acute right ventricular cardiomyopathy referred to as propofol-related infusion syndrome, described in detail in Chapter 4.

Drugs causing dose-dependent cardiac failure

Dose-dependent drug-induced heart failure is classically seen following an overdose of cardiodepressant drugs such as antiarrhythmics and antihypertensives. The two most common drug types associated with circulatory failure are beta blockers and calcium channel antagonists. The negative inotropic and chronotropic effects of beta blockers are well known and mediated directly through the adrenoreceptor pathways. Calcium channel blockers operate by impeding transmembrane calcium flux, a key controlling component of cardiac contractility. In addition, with certain calcium channel blockers such as amlodipine, peripheral arterial vasodilation can accompany this fall in contractility.

Management of beta blocker and calcium channel blocker overdose

Since receptor binding cannot be reversed acutely in either beta blocker or calcium channel blocker overdose, reversal of acute myocardial depression hinges on the myocytes accessing other fuel sources, as shown in Figure 2.25.

During drug-induced shock states, the cardiac myocyte switches its energy source preference from fatty acid to carbohydrate. This metabolic starvation that occurs is exacerbated in calcium channel overdose due to calcium channel-mediated insulin release suppression. In order to maximize the efficiency of the

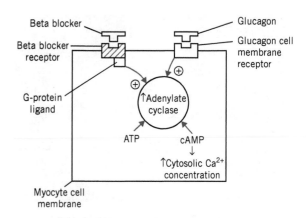

Figure 2.25 Graphical demonstration of the proposed mechanism for glucagon in beta blocker overdose. By stimulating adenylate cyclase via an alternative pathway, the end result of increased cytosolic cyclic adenosine monophosphate (AMP), and therefore calcium, is achieved, despite the classical pathway for intracellular signalling being blocked.

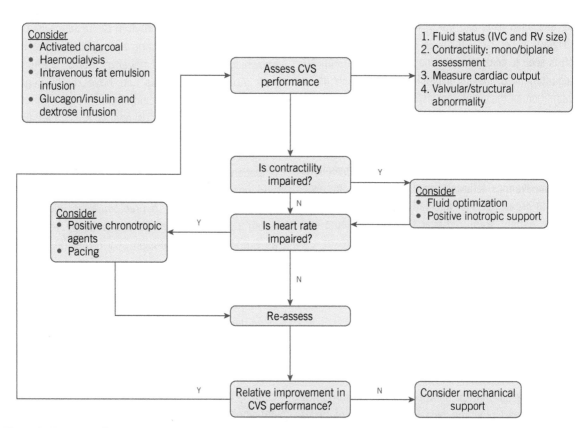

Figure 2.26 Echo-guided assessment and management of the shocked overdose patient.

myocyte, supranormal levels of glucagon and insulin can provide an energy source to allow optimal contractility in the context of drug-induced cardiogenic shock. Administration of glucagon mediates a positive inotropic effect at a cellular level by increasing cytosolic levels of adenylate cyclase. Although initial case reports with glucagon were successful, it is thought this may be an artefact of the manufacturing process. Before biosynthetic techniques were available, bovine glucagon also contained insulin, which is now thought to be the main positive inotropic agent of choice. Current practice remains administration of glucagon primarily, with supplementation of insulin and dextrose subsequently.

Traditional vasoactive medications have limited efficacy in this context, due to the underlying receptor blockade, and often worsen the cardiac output by achieving unwanted vasoconstriction in the setting of impaired contractility. Figure 2.26 describes a practical approach to management of the patient with drug-induced cardiogenic shock.

The management of beta blocker overdose is illustrated in the following case study.

CASE STUDY

How low can you go?—cardiogenic shock secondary to massive beta blocker overdose

A 23-year-old female presented to the emergency department escorted by her mother who reported that her daughter had ingested 5 g of metoprolol with alcohol. On examination, the patient was drowsy, bradycardic (35 bpm), and hypotensive (71/40). The capillary refill time was prolonged at 5 s, and the emergency department had administered 4 L of fluid, with no improvement in her haemodynamics. Arterial blood gas analysis revealed an elevated blood lactate of 3.8. Her Glasgow Coma Score continued to fall to 7, and she was therefore intubated using etomidate and rocuronium. Following intubation, her blood pressure fell further despite boluses of metaraminol and adrenaline. An echocardiogram demonstrated a non-dilated, severely impaired LV and a dilated and impaired RV, with a non-collapsing inferior vena cava (IVC) whilst ventilated. The images are shown in Figure 2.27 ◉ .

An adrenaline infusion was commenced in the emergency department and the patient received a bolus dose of 5 mg of glucagon before being promptly transferred to the intensive

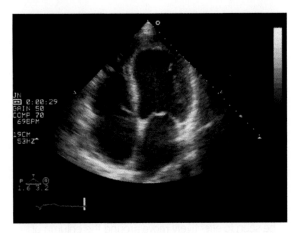

Figure 2.27 [Video 2.14] This apical four-chamber loop demonstrates a globally impaired left ventricle, with a visually estimated ejection fraction that is severely impaired, coupled with an inappropriate bradycardia.

◉ *This video is available to watch in the online video appendix.*

therapy unit. Repeat echocardiography revealed minimal change in left ventricular systolic function despite infusing inotropic support; therefore, a high-dose insulin infusion was commenced, along with glucose and potassium. Repeat imaging revealed mild improvement in systolic function; however, her lactate continued to worsen. The patient was referred for extracorporeal cardiac support and established on veno-arterial extracorporeal circulation for a total of 5 days before being discharged from hospital, having made a complete recovery 2 weeks later. Repeat echocardiography 6 weeks later showed a normal left and right ventricle.

The importance of understanding left ventricular structure

Left ventricular mechanics

The LV is a complex mechanical structure designed to generate a variable SV, depending upon rapidly changing loading conditions. Modern imaging techniques have helped to develop our understanding of the functional anatomy and physiology of this highly developed muscle.

The muscular fibres of the left ventricular wall are arranged in three different planes: radial, longitudinal, and spiral. This muscular array is designed to facilitate synchronous wall contraction at optimal efficiency. Systolic performance is directed towards increasing the total pressure within the LV, such that it exceeds the aortic pressure and generates flow across the aortic valve.

The three planes of left ventricular contraction are appreciated using different components of echocardiographic investigation:

- Radial function is best seen in the parasternal short axis views where thickening of the myocardium can be seen to reduce the end-systolic area by a combination of wall thickening and ejection

- Longitudinal ventricular function is seen best using the apical windows where the base of the heart can be seen to effectively move around the column of blood contained in the heart at the end of diastole and shorten the distance between the base and apex

- Rotational contraction of the LV is the most difficult function to appreciate using standard echocardiographic techniques but is significant to both systolic and diastolic function. The apex and base rotate in opposite directions during systole and diastole and result in a movement analogous to wringing out a wet towel, helping to increase pressure within the ventricle during systole in an apex to outflow tract direction. The resultant unwinding of the LV is also thought to play a role in sucking blood into the LV during early diastole to assist with ventricular filling. Rotation of the apex can be seen, but not measured, using TTE in the apical parasternal short axis view and is a purely qualitative measure of left ventricular function.

Figure 2.28 attempts to demonstrate the wrapping and direction of the three muscular components of the LV.

Left ventricular wall nomenclature

Echocardiography subdivides the LV into regions according to a hybrid of anatomical and arterial territories. When viewing the LV, we refer to three arbitrary levels to subdivide the ventricle in the longitudinal axis:

- Basal at the mitral valve level

- Mid at the mid-papillary muscle level

- Apical to describe the section of the ventricle immediately below the true apex

- On top of these three longitudinal layers sits the true apex, which is a solo ventricular segment, much like the cap placed on top of an igloo.

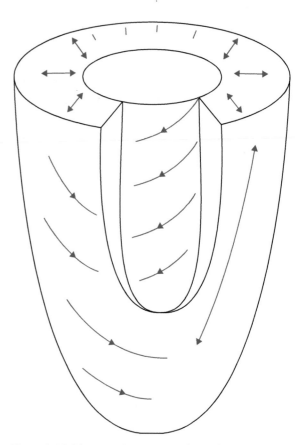

Figure 2.28 Diagram of the myocardial fibrillary alignment within the left ventricle.

The longitudinal levels are then further subclassified into distinct regions according to their position with reference to the RV.

- At the basal and mid-papillary levels, there are six radial segments. The region of the LV that is between the two insertion points of the RV is defined as the septum and incorporates both the antero- and inferoseptal regions, as shown in Figure 2.29.

- The remaining myocardium at the basal and mid-papillary levels is subdivided into four further regions, as shown in Figure 2.29.

- At the level of the apical layer, there is no RV; therefore, the ring of the left ventricular myocardium is subdivided into four distinct areas.

- There are therefore 17 segments of the LV, including the true apex.

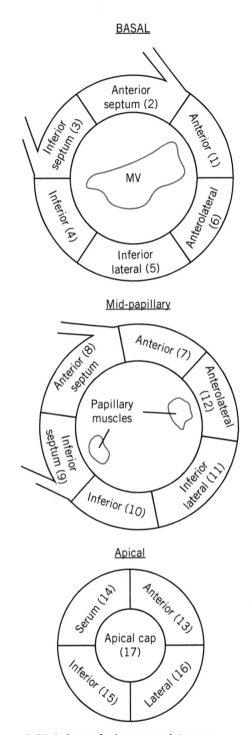

BASAL

Mid-papillary

Apical

Figure 2.29 Left ventricular nomenclature, as demonstrated in the parasternal short axis. Each layer is further subdivided into regions, totalling 17 when the apical cap is included.

Coronary supply to the myocardium

A further method for describing the functional anatomy of the LV is to classify regions according to their arterial perfusion territories. The LV is supplied by a combination of right and left coronary arteries, and significant variations exist; however, the accepted classical format is described graphically in Figure 2.30. By understanding the relationship between arterial supply and regional wall motion abnormalities, the echocardiographer can suggest the arterial location of coronary pathology, but given the variation in arterial supply to the different regions of the myocardium, such assessment remains conjecture until confirmed by angiography.

Left ventricular hypertrophy

Sustained afterload excess results in hyperplasia of the ventricle in order to preserve the EF. Normal myocardial perfusion is derived from two sources—the thin subendocardium receiving blood via diffusion from the ventricular surface, whilst epicardial coronary arteries perfuse the majority of the muscular walls. During systole, these vessels are compressed, resulting in no flow. The greater the muscle bulk, the larger the oxygen demand and the greater the distance the blood must traverse before reaching its destination. Left ventricular hypertrophy (LVH) is therefore strongly associated with ischaemic heart disease.

Hypertrophy can also be the result of abnormal muscle within the ventricle. Several pathological conditions exist where ventricular hypertrophy occurs without a physiological stimulus. Both the distribution of hypertrophy and the appearance of the myocardium can help identify these conditions.

Hypertrophic cardiomyopathy classically causes asymmetrical septal hypertrophy; however, other hypertrophic distributions also exist within this diagnosis. Isolated apical hypertrophy associated with large crypts is a classical feature of non-compaction of the LV. Thought to result from a failure during embryogenesis, the ventricle develops a thick, spongy wall with associated deep crypts or trabeculations, best seen using 2D echocardiography in parasternal and apical views. Right ventricular hypertrophy can be a feature of chronic pulmonary hypertension (PHT) or rarely right ventricular cardiomyopathies such as arrhythmogenic

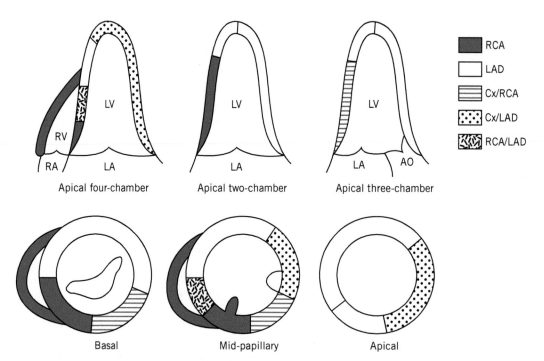

RCA
LAD
Cx/RCA
Cx/LAD
RCA/LAD

Apical four-chamber

Apical two-chamber

Apical three-chamber

Basal

Mid-papillary

Apical

Figure 2.30 Common distribution of epicardial coronary arteries. It is important to note significant variations can occur within these patterns.

right ventricle (hyper-reflective moderator band, trabecular derangement, and sacculations).

Calculation of the relative wall thickness can assist in identifying the likely aetiology of ventricular hypertrophy by assessing for regional variations, and increasingly cardiac magnetic resonance imaging (MRI) is being used in a diagnostic capacity to assist in managing these cohorts.

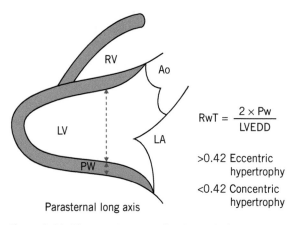

$$RwT = \frac{2 \times Pw}{LVEDD}$$

>0.42 Eccentric hypertrophy

<0.42 Concentric hypertrophy

Parasternal long axis

Figure 2.31 Diagram demonstrating how relative wall thickness can be calculated, assisting in distinguishing between concentric and asymmetrical thickening.

Practice point

Left ventricular structure is relevant to critical illness management, as illustrated in the following case study.

CASE STUDY

Obstructing progress—dynamic outflow tract assessment and obstruction

A 68-year-old male patient was admitted to the intensive care department suffering from septic shock due to ascending cholangitis. Subsequent multi-organ failure was treated with invasive ventilation, broad-spectrum antibiotics, and vasoconstrictor therapy. His previous medical history included hypertension and chronic renal failure. Two weeks later, a tracheostomy was inserted due to prolonged respiratory wean and two failed attempts at extubation. Both attempts at extubation had failed rapidly due to type 1 respiratory failure, which resolved within 48 hours of restarting invasive ventilation and diuretic therapy.

A TTE was performed following his second extubation. The striking abnormalities were moderate concentric LVH and evidence of prolonged left ventricular diastolic deceleration time, in keeping with significant hypertrophy. The left heart was otherwise normal in both structure and function. A repeat echocardiogram performed during a sedation hold and spontaneous breathing trial demonstrated a significant gradient within the LVOT despite the aortic valve opening well.

The echocardiography team concluded that hypertension and tachycardia associated with weaning trials resulted in functional LVOT obstruction due to septal hypertrophy, exacerbated by diuresis. The patient was subsequently treated with beta blockers and vasodilators and was successfully weaned from the ventilator over the next 72 hours. The patient's echocardiographic images are shown in Figures 2.32 and 2.33 📷, and Figures 2.34, 2.35, and 2.36. This group of images begins with the parasternal long axis, showing normal systolic excursion. The notable abnormality is the subaortic ridge, just ventricular of the aortic valve. The next loop demonstrates the turbulence caused by this narrowing within the LVOT, seen as a high-velocity colour signal using colour-flow Doppler in the apical five-chamber view. Doppler analysis of the valvular gradient demonstrates normal transaortic gradients, using continuous wave analysis;

however, when pulsed wave is used to interrogate specific subvalvular regions, a clear subaortic acceleration gradient can be seen to occur as the calliper is advanced towards the aortic valve and site of obstruction.

Regional wall motion abnormalities

Active thickening and inward movement of the myocardium during systole is indicative of a viable myocardium, and the clinician–echocardiographer should use accepted nomenclature to grade the performance of each wall region where this is indicated. The 'regional wall motion score' assigns a value to each of the 17 segments of the myocardium described under 'Left ventricular wall nomenclature', p. 34 to grade global left ventricular performance and monitor changes in regional function. The components of the four-point score are shown in Table 2.2.

Regional wall abnormalities can be subtle, but identifying important regional wall motion impairment is a key component of managing the shocked patient. Chronic regional wall motion abnormalities are associated with myocardial scarring and therefore show

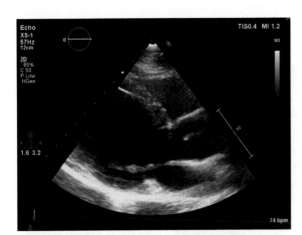

Figure 2.32 [Video 2.15] This parasternal long axis is demonstrating subaortic flow acceleration due to narrowing of the left ventricular outflow tract. This is the product of moderate septal hypertrophy and an elongated anterior mitral valve leaflet which is sucked towards the left ventricular outflow tract during stress states such as extreme tachycardia or hypovolaemia.

📷 *This video is available to watch in the online video appendix.*

© Oxford University Hospitals NHS Foundation Trust 2016, with permission.

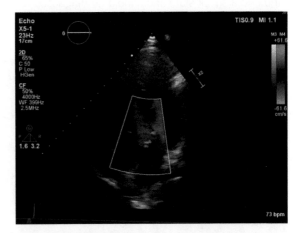

Figure 2.33 [Video 2.16] The apical five-chamber view shows clear subaortic turbulence when colour-flow Doppler is applied to the left ventricular outflow tract region. The change in colour signal is one of the suggestive features that would prompt further spectral Doppler investigation for the presence of subaortic obstruction.

📷 *This video is available to watch in the online video appendix.*

© Oxford University Hospitals NHS Foundation Trust 2016, with permission.

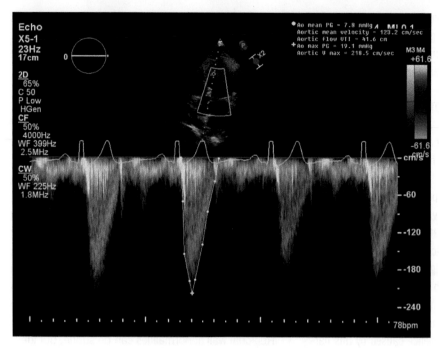

Figure 2.34 Spectral Doppler trace obtained from the apical five-chamber using continuous-wave Doppler. The raised velocity indicates the presence of a raised gradient somewhere along the Doppler pathway, but the location, and therefore aetiology, cannot be identified using this technique alone.

© Oxford University Hospitals NHS Foundation Trust 2016, with permission.

evidence of thinning and calcification of the endocardium. Conversely, hypo- or akinetic regions without these features are more likely to represent recent or current epicardial occlusion. Both findings can contribute to a shock state and should be diagnosed and managed appropriately. The key differences between acute and chronic regional wall motion abnormalities are shown in the following moving images (Figures 2.37 to 2.46 ◉). The images demonstrate the differences between acute and chronic ischaemic

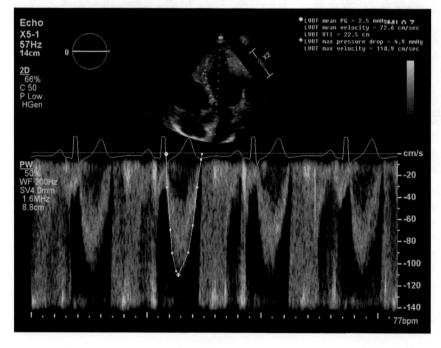

Figure 2.35 Pulsed-wave spectral Doppler trace taken at the level of the subaortic region. This measurement is the location used for normal estimation of aortic valve area gradients and is usually within 1 cm of the aortic valve. This spectral trace shows a raised velocity time integral and peak velocity, suggesting the gradient begins below the valve, rather than within or above, indicating a diagnosis of subaortic flow acceleration.

© Oxford University Hospitals NHS Foundation Trust 2016, with permission.

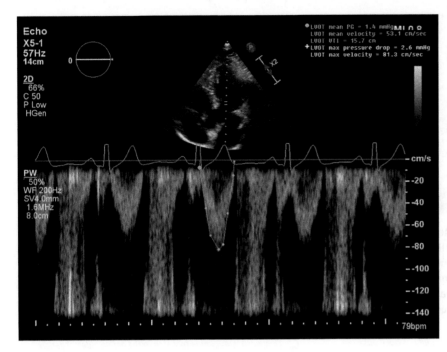

Figure 2.36 Pulsed-wave Doppler trace taken from deeper within the left ventricular cavity reveals a normal-flow acceleration appearance, confirming the diagnosis of subaortic left ventricular outflow tract obstruction. This should prompt investigation to identify the aetiology of the obstruction, along with assessment of the left ventricle for other features indicating a possible cardiomyopathy such as hypertrophic cardiomyopathy.

© Oxford University Hospitals NHS Foundation Trust 2016, with permission.

changes in myocardial appearance. Acute ischaemia has impaired systolic function (hypokinetic or akinetic) but has not atrophied, and may often be hypertrophied as a consequence of risk factors for ischaemic heart disease. In contrast, established infarcted areas of the myocardium are identifiable by the thinned, atrophied regions of the myocardium, often with associated areas of myocardial calcification. Figure 2.38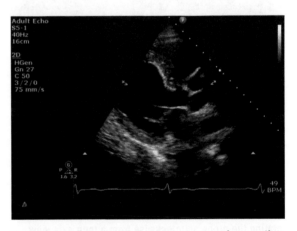

clearly demonstrates a normal-thickness, akinetic septum which is seen in the apical four-chamber to extend down to the apical region. The chronic loops clearly show a calcified, atrophied inferior wall in the

Figure 2.37 [Video 2.17] Parasternal long axis revealing a large akinetic acute regional wall motion abnormality in the septum. The thick, yet akinetic, myocardium points towards an acute event, whilst the marked difference between the septum and the posterior wall indicates a likely coronary aetiology, rather than a global impairment of systolic function such as myocarditis.

This video is available to watch in the online video appendix.

© Oxford University Hospitals NHS Foundation Trust 2016, with permission.

Table 2.2 Components of the RWMA score

Score	Regional myocardial systolic performance
1	Normal
2	Hypokinetic
3	Akinetic
4	Dyskinetic
5	Aneurysmal

RWMA, regional wall motion abnormalities.

The wall motion score index (WMSI) is calculated using the formula: WMSI = sum of all scored regions/total number of regions scored.

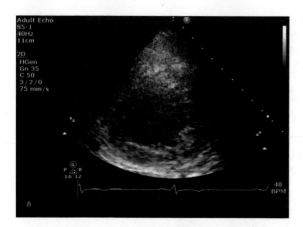

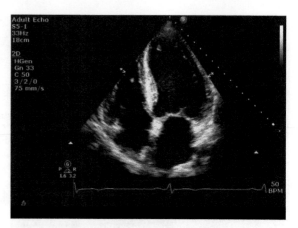

Figure 2.38 [Video 2.18] Parasternal short axis of the same patient at the mid-papillary level. There is preserved systolic function, excluding the inferior and septal walls where the myocardium is akinetic. Again the myocardium has normal appearances, suggesting an acute infarction, rather than chronic established regional abnormalities.

⬤ *This video is available to watch in the online video appendix.*

© Oxford University Hospitals NHS Foundation Trust 2016, with permission.

Figure 2.39 [Video 2.19] This apical four-chamber reveals a large apical regional abnormality with preserved lateral wall systolic function. The overall impact of apical infarcts on the ejection fraction is shown well in this loop and is high risk for developing an apical thrombus as a subacute complication of an acute myocardial infarction.

⬤ *This video is available to watch in the online video appendix.*

© Oxford University Hospitals NHS Foundation Trust 2016, with permission.

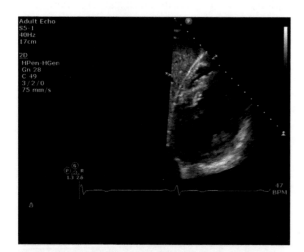

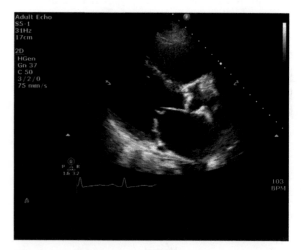

Figure 2.40 [Video 2.20] Subcostal short axis. The same patient viewed via the subcostal axis, achieved by rotating the probe anticlockwise from a long axis view. Often useful in acute situations, this window affords the user the ability to obtain good subcostal views whilst the subject is supine, whilst also allowing assessment of the volume status using the right heart and inferior vena cava.

⬤ *This video is available to watch in the online video appendix.*

© Oxford University Hospitals NHS Foundation Trust 2016, with permission.

Figure 2.41 [Video 2.21] Parasternal long axis with severely impaired systolic function. The left ventricular myocardium is thinned and calcified, in contrast to the appearance in Videos 2.18 and 2.19, suggesting a more established disease course.

⬤ *This video is available to watch in the online video appendix.*

© Oxford University Hospitals NHS Foundation Trust 2016, with permission.

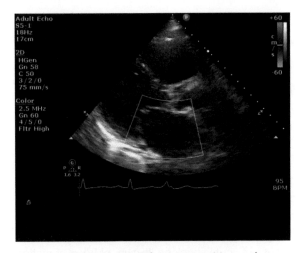

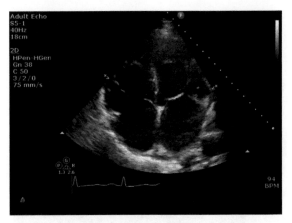

Figure 2.42 [Video 2.22] This parasternal long axis shows the complications of established regional abnormalities within the left ventricle. Mitral valve dysfunction can develop as a chronic consequence of left ventricular dysfunction, either due to posterior mitral valve leaflet dysfunction or dilation of the left ventricle and subsequent failure of the leaflet tips to coapt during ventricular systole.

This video is available to watch in the online video appendix.

© Oxford University Hospitals NHS Foundation Trust 2016, with permission.

Figure 2.43 [Video 2.23] This apical four-chamber shows a thinned and akinetic interventricular septum, suggesting long-standing infarction. The right ventricle is also dilated and impaired, and the biatrial dilation suggests long-standing atrial hypertension, either due to diastolic dysfunction or semilunar regurgitation.

This video is available to watch in the online video appendix.

© Oxford University Hospitals NHS Foundation Trust 2016, with permission.

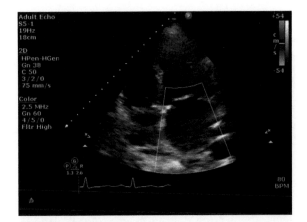

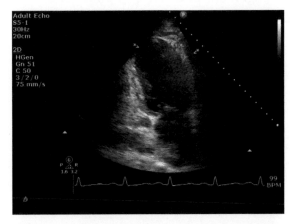

Figure 2.44 [Video 2.24] Apical four-chamber revealing moderate central mitral regurgitation.

This video is available to watch in the online video appendix.

© Oxford University Hospitals NHS Foundation Trust 2016, with permission.

Figure 2.45 [Video 2.25] Apical two-chamber revealing a large chronic regional wall motion abnormality throughout the inferior wall with associated calcification and atrophy.

This video is available to watch in the online video appendix.

© Oxford University Hospitals NHS Foundation Trust 2016, with permission.

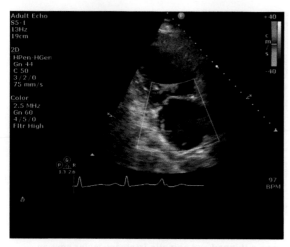

Figure 2.46 [Video 2.26] Apical two-chamber with colour-flow Doppler revealing a moderate jet of central mitral regurgitation.

This video is available to watch in the online video appendix.

© Oxford University Hospitals NHS Foundation Trust 2016, with permission.

apical two-chamber, with significant impairment of systolic function.

Echocardiographic findings and management of acute complications of acute myocardial infarction

Practice point

When assessing a shocked patient who has a probable subacute coronary cause for shock, the following components of the echo exam should be prioritized:

1. Identify and quantify regional wall motion abnormalities and their chronicity
2. Estimate overall left ventricular function
3. Identify ventricular sequelae such as ventriculoseptal defect and left ventricular aneurysm
4. Identify structural and functional abnormalities of the mitral valve and apparatus
5. Assess the function and anatomy of the right heart
6. Exclude inflammation of the pericardium.

Ischaemic pathological sequelae associated with a systolic murmur

Ischaemic mitral regurgitation

Infarction of either the inferolateral or inferior left ventricular wall regions can result in progressive dysfunction of the posterior mitral valve leaflet (pMVL). Calcification and retraction of the supporting apparatus of the pMVL often results in subsequent valve dysfunction. The anterior leaflet will fail to completely coapt with the retracted pMVL, with resultant incompetence of the leaflet and MR directed underneath the anterior mitral valve leaflet (aMVL). This is rarely a cause of acute shock on its own. pMVL dysfunction with subsequent mitral regurgitation is seen in the videos shown in Figures 2.47 to 2.54 . This series of images demonstrates chronic ischaemia and infarction of the basal inferior regions, with subsequent mitral valve dysfunction. The apical two-chamber clearly demonstrates calcification and aneurysmal dilation at the base. Colour-flow Doppler shows two convergent jets of moderate MR. The pMVL is calcified at the base of the leaflet and has restricted mobility shown in the PLAX, whilst the apical four-chamber clearly shows retraction of the pMVL as a consequence of previous ischaemic changes.

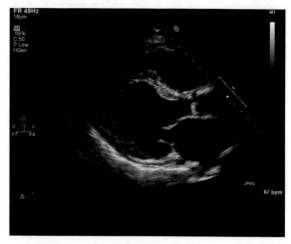

Figure 2.47 [Video 2.27] Parasternal long axis, showing the anterior mitral leaflet opening well but a retracted and relatively immobile posterior leaflet.

This video is available to watch in the online video appendix.

© Oxford University Hospitals NHS Foundation Trust 2016, with permission.

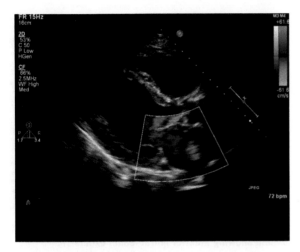

Figure 2.48 [Video 2.28] Parasternal long axis with colour Doppler over the mitral valve, revealing a large jet of mitral regurgitation.

This video is available to watch in the online video appendix.

© Oxford University Hospitals NHS Foundation Trust 2016, with permission.

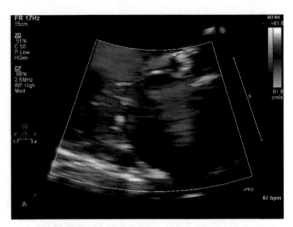

Figure 2.49 [Video 2.29] Zoomed parasternal long axis further detailing the mitral regurgitation.

This video is available to watch in the online video appendix.

© Oxford University Hospitals NHS Foundation Trust 2016, with permission.

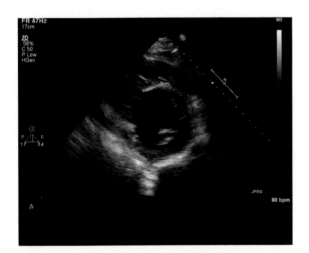

Figure 2.50 [Video 2.30] Parasternal short axis demonstrating preserved radial function of the left ventricle after primary coronary intervention.

This video is available to watch in the online video appendix.

© Oxford University Hospitals NHS Foundation Trust 2016, with permission.

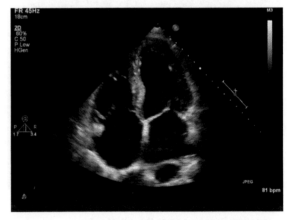

Figure 2.51 [Video 2.31] Apical four-chamber revealing retracted and immobile posterior mitral valve leaflet.

This video is available to watch in the online video appendix.

© Oxford University Hospitals NHS Foundation Trust 2016, with permission.

Papillary muscle or chordal rupture

The subvalvular structure of the mitral valve is anchored by the inferoseptal and anterolateral papillary muscles, as shown in Figure 2.55. Chordae then attach from the papillary muscles to the undersurface of the mitral valve leaflets.

The subvalvular apparatus operates to prevent prolapse of the mitral leaflets into the atrium during ventricular systole. Conventionally, the inferoseptal muscle receives its arterial blood supply from the right coronary artery and the anterolateral papillary muscle from the circumflex artery. Acute interruption of the

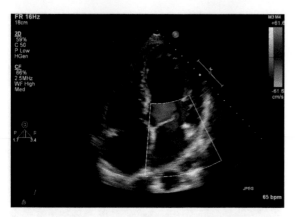

Figure 2.52 [Video 2.32] Colour-flow Doppler of the apical four-chamber further demonstrating mitral regurgitation.

📹 *This video is available to watch in the online video appendix.*

© Oxford University Hospitals NHS Foundation Trust 2016, with permission.

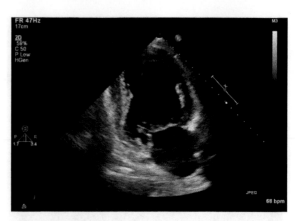

Figure 2.53 [Video 2.33] Apical two-chamber of the same patient showing anterior mitral leaflet excursion.

📹 *This video is available to watch in the online video appendix.*

© Oxford University Hospitals NHS Foundation Trust 2016, with permission.

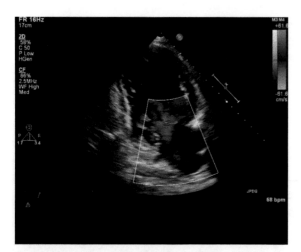

Figure 2.54 [Video 2.34] Apical two-chamber with colour-flow Doppler across the mitral valve, completing the assessment of the mitral valve. The atrial dilation points towards a chronic, rather than acute, pathology.

📹 *This video is available to watch in the online video appendix.*

© Oxford University Hospitals NHS Foundation Trust 2016, with permission.

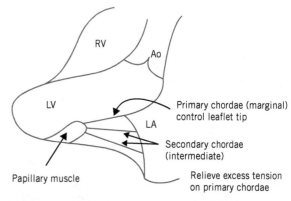

Figure 2.55 Diagram of the papillary muscles and chordae connections to the mitral valve leaflets, demonstrating the chordae bridging from the papillary muscle to the relevant insertion on the ventricular aspect of the valve.

arterial supply to the papillary muscles can result in rupture or dysfunction of the subvalvular structure and subsequent acute left ventricular failure due to flail or prolapse of the mitral valve leaflets. An example of a flail pMVL is seen in the clip shown in Figures 2.56 to 2.60 📹. Acute chordal rupture can also present in a similar, although often less severe, shock state. Flail pMVL is clearly demonstrated in the PLAX, with the leaflet tip prolapsing into the atria during ventricular systole with associated anteriorly directed severe MR shown in the colour Doppler loops in PLAX and apical four-chamber. The atria are mildly dilated, suggesting that this is an acute complication following damage to the mitral subvalvular apparatus. Systolic ventricular performance appears hyperdynamic; however, interpretation must acknowledge the significant retrograde

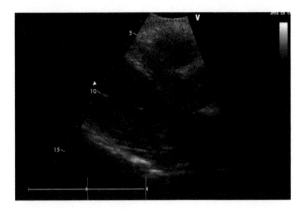

Figure 2.56 [Video 2.35] Parasternal long axis showing opening of the mitral valve.

🎥 *This video is available to watch in the online video appendix.*

© Oxford University Hospitals NHS Foundation Trust 2016, with permission.

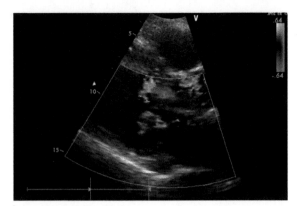

Figure 2.57 [Video 2.36] Parasternal long axis with colour-flow Doppler across the mitral valve revealing the mitral regurgitation.

🎥 *This video is available to watch in the online video appendix.*

© Oxford University Hospitals NHS Foundation Trust 2016, with permission.

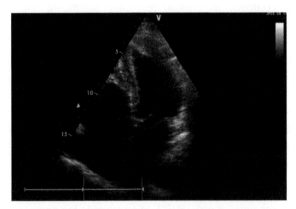

Figure 2.58 [Video 2.37] Apical four-chamber showing prolapse of the anterior mitral valve leaflet into the left atrial cavity following destruction of the sub valvular architecture.

🎥 *This video is available to watch in the online video appendix.*

© Oxford University Hospitals NHS Foundation Trust 2016, with permission.

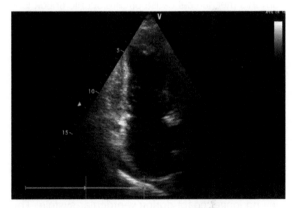

Figure 2.59 [Video 2.38] Apical two-chamber further demonstrating prolapse of the anterior leaflet into the left atrium.

🎥 *This video is available to watch in the online video appendix.*

© Oxford University Hospitals NHS Foundation Trust 2016, with permission.

shunt into the atria during systole, masking any possible systolic dysfunction.

Patients with papillary muscle rupture present with a mixture of shock and acute, often profound, pulmonary oedema. The extreme acuity of the MR causes a sudden rise in LVEDP to which the right heart has had no time to adapt.

Echocardiographically, the affected leaflet tip will be seen to pass beyond the horizontal axis of the mitral valve annulus, and colour-flow Doppler will demonstrate a jet of MR directed away from the prolapsing leaflet. The jet is often eccentric and requires several views to accurately quantify its severity. The basal parasternal short axis view can help in identifying the exact location of the prolapse and assist in surgical planning. Management is with immediate intubation to reduce the work of breathing and provide positive end-expiratory pressure (PEEP) to combat the raised LVEDP. Mortality

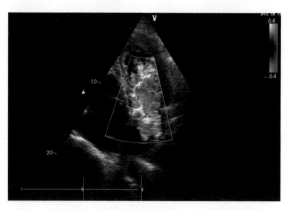

Figure 2.60 [Video 2.39] Colour flow across the mitral valve further demonstrating the acute mitral regurgitation into the left atrium.

This video is available to watch in the online video appendix.
© Oxford University Hospitals NHS Foundation Trust 2016, with permission.

from this mechanical cause of cardiogenic shock is in excess of 70%. Definitive management requires rapid identification and surgical intervention.

Left ventricular dilatation and functional mitral regurgitation

This is rarely the cause of a systolic murmur in acute myocardial infarction (MI) without a previous history of infarction or cardiac comorbidity such as ischaemic or alcoholic cardiomyopathy. Dilatation of the LV gradually pulls the mitral valve tips apart until they no longer coapt during ventricular systole. This results in central MR of varying severity. To make this diagnosis, the valve architecture should be otherwise normal and the LV above the normal cavity size in diastole.

Acute ventriculoseptal defect

Infarction affecting the interventricular septum can result in such extensive necrosis that the integrity of the wall is compromised. This complication of myocardial ischaemia classically occurs at day 3 post-infarction. The necrotic area allows communication between the two ventricles, with flow classically occurring from left to right owing to the interventricular pressure gradient. The septum is broadly split into two regions referred to as membranous and muscular. The membranous septum is located adjacent to the basal septal region and forms part of the LVOT. The

muscular section of the septum forms the remaining wall. Ischaemic ventricular septal defects are classically encountered within the muscular septum and are often multiple and can be small. They are more commonly found in association following anterior infarction (60%); however, they are a recognized complication of posteroinferior infarction and may present with associated mitral valve dysfunction. Ventricular septal defects are best viewed using either parasternal short axis or apical four-chamber views using colour-flow Doppler to identify a left-to-right shunt. Placing the colour box across the septum in the short axis and gradually scanning along the length of the ventricle right up to the apex where a ventriculoseptal defect can easily be missed is a robust technique. The subcostal view is also very helpful when looking for a ventriculoseptal defect. Dilation of the RV and possible associated tricuspid regurgitation (TR) may accompany a haemodynamically significant shunt and should be examined for.

Aneurysm

Seen in approximately 5% of patients following an MI, ventricular aneurysms are associated with a poor prognosis. Left ventricular aneurysms are subclassified into true and false aneurysms, according to their structure.

- True aneurysms are most commonly located within the anterior wall (80%), often towards the apex. They have a wide neck and their walls are entirely composed of myocardium.

- False aneurysms are usually located in the inferior and inferolateral territories and have a narrow neck. False aneurysms are actually areas of full-thickness necrosis of the left ventricular wall with subsequent flow of blood into a contained area within the pericardium. Uncontained false aneurysms present as tamponade and sudden death usually 3 days following an MI.

To distinguish them, colour-flow imaging will demonstrate either absent or swirling blood flow patterns within true aneurysms, whilst a clear pulsatile colour flow will be seen in and out of false aneurysms in sync with contraction of the LV. The likely cause of a cardiac aneurysm is ischaemic; however, there is a differential diagnosis which includes cardiac sarcoidosis, Chagas' disease, and congenital causes. Figure 2.61 illustrates the identifying differences between a true and false aneurysm.

Thrombus

Akinetic inflamed regions of the myocardium act as prothrombotic generators, and thrombus formation is a well-recognized subacute complication of MI within the damaged territory. The classical echocardiographic features of a thrombus are a high-density structure overlying an akinetic cardiac segment. Classically, a cleavage plane is described, related to the interface between the endocardium and the clot. Contrast administration may assist in delineating potential clots. As with any potential intracardiac mass, its existence is confirmed by demonstrating the thrombus using multiple views, as well as measuring and grading the relevant mobility of the thrombus. The moving image shown in Figure 2.62 ▭ demonstrates an apical thrombus with classical hyperdensity, cleavage plane, and mobility related to wall contraction, overlying large regional wall motion abnormalities. Apical four-chamber demonstrating a large apical akinetic regional wall motion abnormality, with associated intraventricular thrombus. Features suggestive of a thrombus are adjacent regional wall motion abnormalities, cleavage plane, and hyperdensity within the left ventricular chamber. Although this thrombus

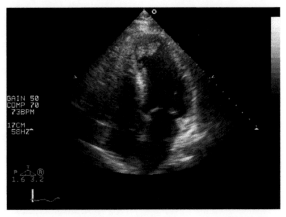

Figure 2.62 [Video 2.40] Apical four-chamber revealing a fixed, echogenic mass located at the apex of the left ventricle. The associated regional impairment of the apex of the left ventricle makes a thrombus a high likelihood.

▭ *This video is available to watch in the online video appendix.*
© Oxford University Hospitals NHS Foundation Trust 2016, with permission.

appears relatively fixed, assessment of mobility must be incorporated. Suspicion of thrombi can often be clarified with the administration of sonographic contrast.

Takotsubo's cardiomyopathy

Takotsubo's cardiomyopathy is an unusual and characteristic regional wall motion abnormality, which is non-ischaemic in aetiology. The origin of Takotsubo is in reference to the shape the LV creates, which is similar to squid traps used in Japan.

The classical description of a Takotsubo's cardiomyopathic LV is normal basal radial function with dilatation and impairment of the apical segments and a variable effect of the mid-papillary regions. This apical ballooning is of unknown aetiology but may represent tachyphylaxis of adrenoreceptors, which are not uniformly distributed throughout the myocardium. This cardiomyopathy can be seen following massive adrenergic surge, for example following subarachnoid haemorrhage, and is most commonly found in postmenopausal women. Angiography within this cohort is characteristically normal. Variants exist, with 'reverse Takotsubo' affecting the basal regions in the context of preserved apical function. Management is supportive, with focus being on restoration of adequate, but

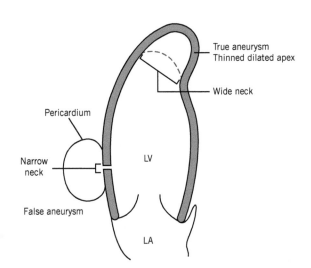

Figure 2.61 Illustration identifying the significant differences between true and false aneurysms.

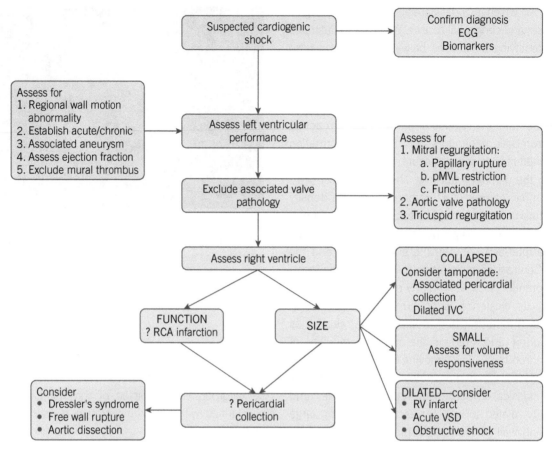

Figure 2.63 **Systematic approach to the investigation of shock with presumed cardiogenic cause.**

not normal, cardiac output using inotropes and consideration of support devices such as balloon pumps or assist devices. In-hospital mortality is low but increases significantly in males or if the presentation was in the context of another critical illness such as sepsis or acute kidney injury.

Dressler's syndrome

Also known as post-MI syndrome, the combination of:

- Low-grade fever
- Pleuritic chest pain and
- Features associated with pericardial effusion

is seen in 5–10% of patients between 2 and 10 weeks post-infarction. Thought to stem from autoantigen expression by an infarcted myocardium, the key echocardiographic component of assessment of suspected

Dressler's is the presence and consequence of any pericardial collection. Although rare, tamponade can occur and conclusive evidence documenting its presence or absence is essential.

Figure 2.63 can be used to comprehensively assess the shocked patient with a possible complication of ischaemic heart disease.

CASE STUDY

Plucking heart strings—acute heart failure following mechanical valve failure

A 73-year-old male was admitted to the ICU following a witnessed out-of-hospital cardiac arrest. He had been feeling unwell for several days at home before attempting to contact his doctor. His history included treated hypertension and diabetes and stable angina. The initial rhythm was ventricular fibrillation which responded to a brief period of advanced life support and defibrillation. The ECG in the resuscitation room revealed obvious inferior and anterior changes which prompted emergency coronary angiography, with some moderate proximal flow obstruction treated with stent insertion. Post-procedure, he was transferred to the ICU, intubated and ventilated to facilitate a period of controlled temperature management and optimization of his post-cardiac arrest syndrome. Ten days later, his cardiac support and sedation had been weaned successfully and was requiring minimal respiratory support, prompting a trial of extubation.

Post-extubation, he rapidly desaturated despite high-flow oxygen and physiotherapy. He was reintubated within 2 hours and required high levels of PEEP to maintain adequate oxygenation. Twelve hours later, his respiratory support requirement had rapidly fallen, which prompted an echocardiogram to assess left ventricular function and identify causes of possible pulmonary oedema.

Following discussion with cardiology, he was slowly weaned from positive pressure ventilation, whilst his heart failure medication was optimized, before being extubated to non-invasive ventilation (NIV). Despite maximal heart failure therapy, the patient was unable to wean from positive pressure ventilation, and therefore surgical repair of the aMVL was successfully performed (Figures 2.64 to 2.68 ▣). The parasternal long axis demonstrates clear flailing of the aMVL with associated severe MR. Post-angiogram, the

systolic function of the myocardium is normal, with no clear regional wall motion abnormality shown in any of the loops.

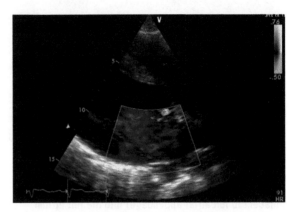

Figure 2.65 [Video 2.42] Use of colour-flow Doppler in the parasternal long axis to demonstrate severe mitral regurgitation following the flail prolapse of the anterior mitral valve leaflet. A small coexisting jet of aortic regurgitation is seen at the top of the colour-flow window in the same loop.

🎥 *This video is available to watch in the online video appendix.*

© Oxford University Hospitals NHS Foundation Trust 2016, with permission.

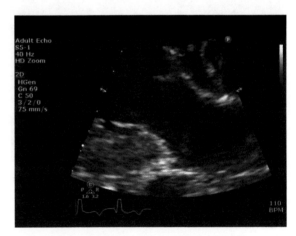

Figure 2.66 [Video 2.43] This image is an apical four-chamber of the same patient, showing abnormal movement of the anterior mitral valve leaflet in both atrial and ventricular systole. The anterior mitral valve leaflet tip is seen to flail within the left ventricular cavity during atrial systole, whilst the leaflet tip can be seen to prolapse within the atrial cavity during ventricular systole. The right ventricle is normal in size and function, and the relatively normal size of the left atrium points towards an acute, rather than chronic, aetiology.

🎥 *This video is available to watch in the online video appendix.*

© Oxford University Hospitals NHS Foundation Trust 2016, with permission.

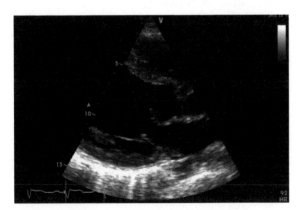

Figure 2.64 [Video 2.41] This shows abnormal hyperdynamic movement of the aMVL with prolapse of the tips into the left atrium during ventricular systole. The left ventricular systolic function is normal, although this must be interpreted in the context of coexisting likely severe mitral regurgitation.

🎥 *This video is available to watch in the online video appendix.*

© Oxford University Hospitals NHS Foundation Trust 2016, with permission.

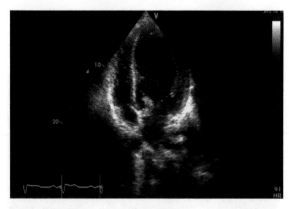

Figure 2.67 [Video 2.44] This image clearly shows the A2 leaflet of the anterior mitral valve leaflet prolapsing at its coaption point with P3 (left side) and P1 (right side, adjacent to left atrial appendage) into the left atrium. Again, the relatively normal left atrial size points towards an acute pathology, especially when the severity of the mitral regurgitation is taken into account.

📷 *This video is available to watch in the online video appendix.*

© Oxford University Hospitals NHS Foundation Trust 2016, with permission.

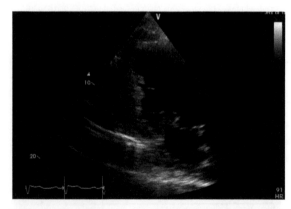

Figure 2.68 [Video 2.45] A zoomed parasternal long axis performed on the day of surgery, further demonstrating full prolapse of the anterior mitral valve leaflet into the left atrium.

📷 *This video is available to watch in the online video appendix.*

© Oxford University Hospitals NHS Foundation Trust 2016, with permission.

Multiple choice questions

1. When assessing left ventricular systolic function, the following are considered independent of loading conditions:
   A Simpson's ejection fraction
   B Visual eyeball
   C Tei index
   D dP/dT
   E Fractional shortening

2. The following are true for false ventricular aneurysms:
   A Classically occur early
   B Wide-necked
   C Common
   D Are often fatal
   E Occur apically commonly

3. The following are recognized direct causes of cardiogenic shock in overdose:
   A Paracetamol
   B Verapamil
   C Insulin
   D Digoxin
   E Bupropion

4. The following techniques provide biplane estimates of ejection fraction:
   A Fractional shortening
   B Simpson's
   C Area length technique
   D Bullet formula
   E MAPSE

5. Acute myocardial ischaemia is favoured in the presence of:
   A Hypokinetic calcified myocardial territories
   B Normal-sized left atrium associated with flail mitral leaflet movement
   C True apical aneurysm
   D Atrial septal defect
   E Pericardial effusion

For answers to multiple choice questions, please see 'Appendix 1: Answers to multiple choice questions', p. 171.

Further reading

Bergenzaun L, Gudmundsson P, Öhlin H, *et al*. Assessing left ventricular systolic function in shock: evaluation of echocardiographic parameters in intensive care. *Crit Care* 2011; 15: R200.

Leeson P, Mitchell ARJ, Becher H. *Echocardiography* (Oxford Specialist Handbook in Cardiology). Oxford University Press, Oxford, 2007.

Newton J, Sabharwal N, Myerson SG, Westaby S, Prendergast B. *Valvular Heart Disease* (Oxford Specialist Handbooks in Cardiology). Oxford University Press, Oxford, 2011.

Otto CM. *Textbook of Clinical Echocardiography*, fifth edition. Elsevier Saunders, Philadelphia, 2013.

Repessé X, Charron C, Vieillard-Baron A. Evaluation of left ventricular systolic function revisited in septic shock. *Crit Care* 2013; **17**: 164.

Vieillard-Baron A. Septic cardiomyopathy. *Ann Intensive Care* 2011; **1**: 6.

3

Interpretation and implication of diastolic dysfunction in critically ill patients

Diastole—the 'other half'

Clinical interest in heart failure in critically ill patients has predominantly focused on systolic dysfunction since Maclean described a group of patients in septic shock with a low cardiac output state in the 1960s. Diastolic dysfunction is common in the critically ill patient population both as a pre-existing disease state and as a consequence of critical illness, but it has been relatively less investigated. Over half of patients who present to the emergency department with cardiogenic pulmonary oedema have normal systolic function. Diastolic dysfunction in critical illness may carry an independent mortality effect and has a significant impact on diagnosis and optimal patient management.

Diastole and the cardiac cycle

The earliest description of diastole was made by Leonardo Da Vinci: 'the atria or filling chambers contract together while the pumping chambers or ventricles are relaxing'.

The LV needs to cycle between two anatomical states during each single heart beat in order to carry out two different functions. During diastole, the LV becomes compliant to allow filling from a low left atrial pressure; during systole, it is a stiff chamber that allows it to eject this volume of blood at arterial pressures (Figure 3.1). Mechanistically, diastole occurs between closure of the mitral valve and opening of the aortic valve. Physiologically, it encompasses four processes (or phases) that occur in the period of time during which

the myocardium loses its ability to generate force and returns to an unstressed pressure and myocyte length. The four phases are shown in Figure 3.2, along with pressure changes in the left atrium (LA) and LV.

- **Phase I—isovolumetric relaxation**: this first phase is energy-dependent, taking place prior to the opening of the mitral valve. Adenosine triphosphate (ATP) is required to break the actin–myosin cross-bridges. The intracardiac pressure drops to its lowest point at the end of this phase (the minimal LV diastolic pressure).
- **Phase II—early filling**: the second phase accounts for up to 80% of ventricular filling. The low resting pressure within the left ventricular cavity facilitates the easy flow of blood from the LA into the ventricle.
- **Phase III—diastasis**: the third phase describes the equalization of left atrial and left ventricular pressures and is very short or non-existent at very high heart rates.
- **Phase IV—atrial systole**: the fourth phase of diastole occurs as the atria contract to fill the ventricle with the final 10–20% of the total end-diastolic volume. This phase is absent during atrial fibrillation (AF), resulting in loss of the 'atrial kick'.

Diastolic dysfunction

In health, isovolumetric relaxation leads to a minimal left ventricular diastolic pressure that is low enough to create a suction effect. This promotes left ventricular

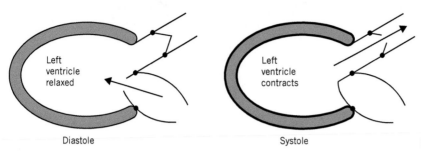

Diastole   Systole

Figure 3.1 **The cardiac cycle.**

filling, resulting in an adequate end-diastolic volume without an increase in left atrial pressure, both at rest and during exercise.

Diastolic dysfunction is an abnormality of left ventricular distensibility, filling, or relaxation, irrespective of systolic function.

If the active relaxation and/or the passive elastic properties of the LV are impaired, then the resting diastolic pressure within the left ventricular cavity will rise. The gradient between the LA and LV falls, reducing passive blood flow into the LV during the second phase of diastole. The left atrial pressure and volume will start to increase to maintain left ventricular filling, resulting in a switch from 'left ventricular pull' to 'left atrial push'. Figure 3.3 shows the pressure changes between phase I and phase II of diastole, both in health (on the left) and where the minimal left ventricular diastolic pressure is increased (on the right).

Heart failure with a normal ejection fraction (HFNEF) describes the clinical syndrome of left ventricular failure with a normal EF and is due to underlying diastolic dysfunction. In HFNEF, the symptoms and signs of heart failure develop as a consequence of the elevation in left-sided filling pressures, leading to pulmonary

venous congestion, pulmonary oedema, and a reduction in lung compliance. High sympathetic drive further reduces the time available for diastolic filling by increasing the heart rate, which, in turn, leads to a low SV despite a normal EF. These cardiopulmonary pressure changes are shown in Figure 3.4.

> **Practice point**
>
> Diastole is an equal partner to systole.
>
> Failure of diastolic processes can present with pulmonary oedema, even where systolic function is normal.

Assessment of diastolic function in non-critically ill patients

Left heart catheterization is the reference method for the assessment of diastolic dysfunction. The pressure monitor at the tip of the catheter measures the resting pressure in the LV directly—the LVEDP. Pulmonary capillary wedge pressures obtained during right heart catheterization can be used as a surrogate measure, but this method assumes there are no further pressure changes between the LA and the pulmonary artery (PA; which is rarely the case in critical illness). TTE can accurately assess the degree and cause of diastolic dysfunction non-invasively at the bedside and has replaced invasive measurement in both cardiology practice and critical care.

Qualitative echocardiographic signs of diastolic function

- If LVH is present, it is highly likely that there will be a degree of diastolic dysfunction. LVH impairs relaxation, reducing early passive filling.

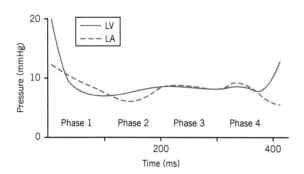

Figure 3.2 **The four phases of the cardiac cycle.**

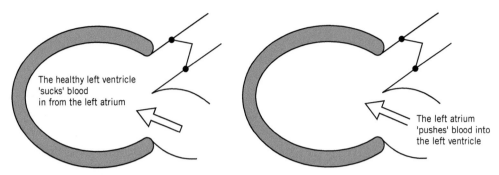

Figure 3.3 **Changes in left-sided pressures in diastolic dysfunction.**

- Left atrial volume reflects the effect of raised left ventricular filling pressure over time. In the absence of left-sided valve disease or inter-atrial shunt, left atrial volume reflects an elevation of LVEDP from either systolic or diastolic dysfunction.

- The inter-atrial septum can bulge towards the right atrium. In health, the inter-atrial septum moves gently to and fro, reflecting the cycling pressures in the atrium during the cardiac cycle. As the left atrial pressure rises, the septum will first remain in a fixed position throughout the cardiac cycle and then bulge consistently towards the right atrium.

- Patients with diastolic dysfunction often have raised PA pressures. Therefore, in the absence of primary pulmonary disease, increased PA pressures can be used to infer elevated left ventricular filling pressures. Common echocardiographic methods to look for PHT include measurement of the right ventricular systolic pressure (RVSP) in patients with TR, the mean and diastolic PA pressure in patients with pulmonary regurgitation (PR), and the pulmonary acceleration time (PAT).

Quantitative echocardiographic measures of diastolic dysfunction

Transmitral Doppler patterns

Assessment of blood flow across the mitral valve is performed using pulsed-wave Doppler. Figure 3.5 demonstrates the phases of left ventricular filling during diastole where the patient is in sinus rhythm.

- The first wave is the E wave and represents passive movement of blood across the mitral valve into the LV during phase II of the diastolic cycle. In health, this accounts for the majority of filling.

- The second wave is the A wave and represents active atrial contraction in phase IV of the diastolic

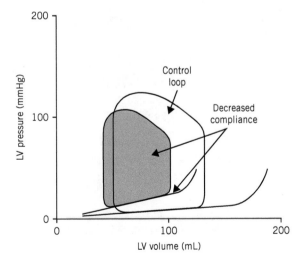

Figure 3.4 **Left ventricular pressure–volume loop.**

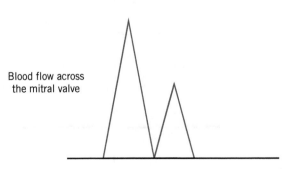

Figure 3.5 **Pulsed-wave Doppler across the mitral valve.**

cycle, accounting for 10–20% of left ventricular filling in health.

From this, we can obtain:

- The peak E wave velocity
- The peak A wave velocity
- The ratio of the E/A waves
- The time taken for passive filling to decelerate from peak to zero—the DT.

These four key measures are shown in Figure 3.6. They alter in characteristic patterns to reflect a rise in the LVEDP.

Pulsed-wave transmitral Doppler is used in the apical four-chamber view, with a 1- to 3-mm sample volume placed between the mitral leaflet tips. Colour-flow imaging can be used to ensure optimal alignment of the Doppler beam at the point of mitral leaflet coaptation. The sweep speed should initially be set to 25–50 mm/s to look for flow variation with respiration. If this is not present, the sweep speed should be increased to 100 mm/s, and the waveform should be taken at end-expiration and averaged over three consecutive cycles. Correct positioning of the pulsed-wave Doppler beam is shown in Figure 3.7.

Current guidelines for the assessment of diastolic dysfunction identify four patterns of mitral inflow:

- Normal
- Grade I diastolic dysfunction: impaired relaxation
- Grade II diastolic dysfunction: pseudonormalization (the E/A ratio returns to normal as a result of a compensatory increase in the left atrial pressure)
- Grade III diastolic dysfunction: restrictive filling.

These patterns and the accompanying diagnostic ranges of E, A, E/A, and DT are shown in Figure 3.8. Transmitral Doppler does not provide a complete picture, for example one cannot differentiate normal from pseudonormal transmitral Doppler patterns, and patients in AF have no A wave. We therefore need to add two further measures to our assessment of diastolic dysfunction: pulmonary venous flow patterns and tissue Doppler assessment of the mitral valve annulus.

Pulmonary venous flow

The pulmonary veins drain into the LA, and blood flow is normally forwards in both systole and diastole, with a short retrograde period of flow during atrial contraction.

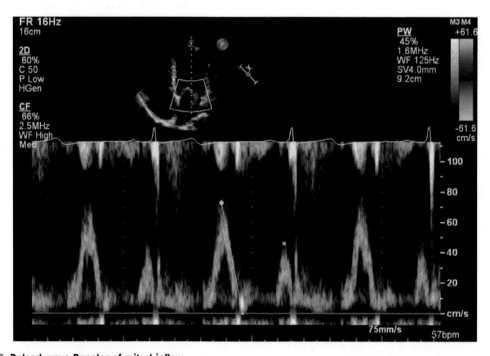

Figure 3.6 Pulsed-wave Doppler of mitral inflow.
© Oxford University Hospitals NHS Foundation Trust 2016, with permission.

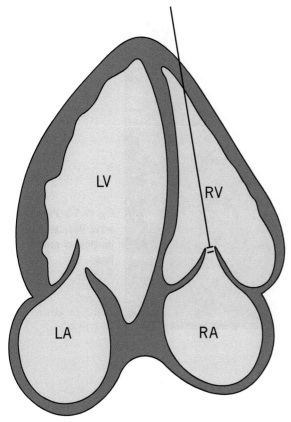

Figure 3.7 Positioning of the pulsed-wave Doppler beam for mitral inflow.

- The S wave represents blood flow into the pulmonary veins during right ventricular systole.

- The D wave represents blood flow during the passive period of left ventricular diastole.

- The a wave occurs during atrial contraction.

These three waves are shown in their normal pattern in Figure 3.9.

From this pattern, we can measure:

- The S/D ratio: in normality, the systolic wave is dominant; as left ventricular filling pressure rises, this wave flattens and the diastolic wave becomes dominant.

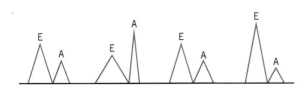

Figure 3.8 The four patterns of mitral inflow.

- The peak a velocity: this is usually low and increases with rising LVEDP.

- The a wave duration (a dur): usually short; this lengthens with increasing LVEDP.

Figure 3.10 demonstrates the changes in the pattern of pulmonary venous flow seen with increasing LVEDP.

The pulmonary venous flow pattern begins to change significantly as the patient approaches grade II diastolic dysfunction, and it is therefore most useful when pseudonormalization is suspected.

Pulmonary venous flow patterns are examined using pulsed-wave Doppler placed approximately 0.5 cm inside the entrance of the pulmonary veins in the apical four-chamber view (Figure 3.11). Colour flow imaging is often used to guide positioning. Any of the pulmonary veins can be used, but the right upper pulmonary vein is often the most accessible. Recordings should be obtained at end-expiration with a sweep speed of 50–100 ms, averaged over three consecutive cycles where there is significant beat-to-beat variability.

Caveats to interpreting pulmonary venous Doppler patterns are:

- In patients with a reduced EF, a reduced systolic fraction of >40% is related to an increase in left atrial pressure due to **systolic dysfunction**

- The a–A duration is the time difference between the duration of the a wave and the duration of the mitral inflow A wave, and is a reliable age- and EF-independent predictor of increased LVEDP.

Practice point

Interpreting pulmonary venous flow patterns relies upon a clean Doppler trace and should not be overinterpreted either as a lone marker of diastolic dysfunction or where the trace is poor.

Tissue Doppler annular velocities

The second technique which we can use to examine diastolic function, in addition to the key information obtained from transmitral Doppler, is TDi. In contrast to blood velocity imaging using conventional Doppler, tissue Doppler specifically looks at the low-velocity

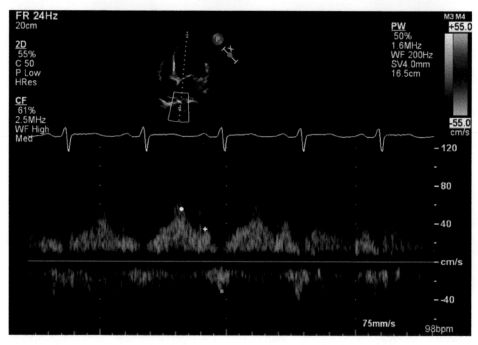

Figure 3.9 **Pulsed-wave Doppler of pulmonary venous flow.**
© Oxford University Hospitals NHS Foundation Trust 2016, with permission.

movements of the ventricular walls and can add information about active relaxation where we need to differentiate normal from pseudonormal function and where the patient is in AF.

TDi is performed using a sample volume of pulsed-wave Doppler placed over the basal part of the left ventricular wall either medially or laterally where the mitral annulus inserts in the apical four-chamber view. The sample volume is placed within 1 cm of both the septal and lateral insertion sites of the mitral leaflets (Figure 3.12). The velocity scale should be around 20 cm/s above and below the zero velocity baseline. Recordings should be obtained at a sweep speed of 50–100 mm/s at end-expiration, averaged over three consecutive cardiac cycles.

Tissue Doppler actively filters out high-velocity signals from the moving red blood cells and displays the low-velocity signals obtained from the annular movement of the LV. Figure 3.13 shows the typical waveform obtained and the labelled individual peaks.

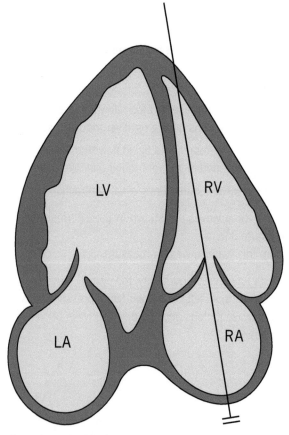

Figure 3.11 **Positioning of the pulsed-wave Doppler beam for pulmonary venous flow.**

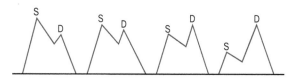

Figure 3.10 **The four patterns of pulmonary venous flow.**

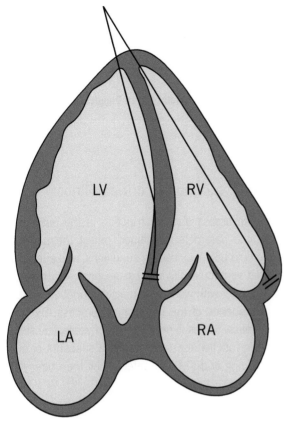

Figure 3.12 Positioning of the pulsed-wave Doppler beam for tissue Doppler imaging.

- The early diastolic velocity is known as e′ ('e-prime') and represents active relaxation of the ventricle.
- It can be thought of as a mirror image of transmitral blood flow into the ventricle during the E wave. In health, it occurs around 20 ms earlier and hence provides a suction effect for the E wave. In diastolic dysfunction, it occurs at the same time as, or later than, the E wave (filling is then more passive).
- Studies have shown that e′ is a load-independent marker of left ventricular relaxation.
- In practice, the average of the lateral or medial annular velocities should be used, and the focus should be on producing a clean waveform.
- As the resting LVEDP rises, the e′ wave shortens.
- The late diastolic velocity is known as a′ ('a-prime') and represents myocardial velocity associated with atrial contraction.

Figure 3.14 shows the progressive reduction in the height of the e′ wave as we progress through the grades of diastolic dysfunction.

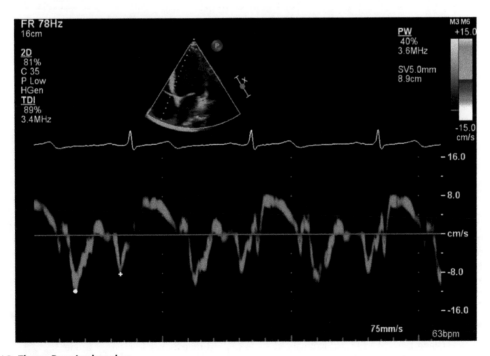

Figure 3.13 Tissue Doppler imaging.

© Oxford University Hospitals NHS Foundation Trust 2016, with permission.

Practice point

- e′ describes the compliance of the LV in a load-independent manner.
- By measuring both the E and e′ wave velocities, we can calculate the E/e′ ratio.
- An E/e′ ratio <8 is associated with normal left ventricular filling pressures.
- An E/e′ ratio >13 is associated with increased filling pressures.
- Values between 8 and 13 represent a grey area and highlight the fact that diastolic function should be assessed using as many qualitative and quantitative markers as possible.

Combining the parameters to assess diastolic function

Figure 3.15 combines the indices described previously to make an assessment of diastolic function.

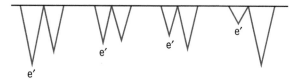

Figure 3.14 Mitral annular tissue Doppler.

Diastolic function in critical illness

When we assess diastolic function in the outpatient clinic, the parameters obtained reflect the patient's stable fluid balance, loading conditions, and afterload. The left ventricular filling pressure rises in a predictable manner with worsening diastolic function, as it is a consequence of the pathological process. By contrast, critical illness is not a steady physiological state. Diastolic functional assessment is a snapshot of current loading and afterload affected by the underlying

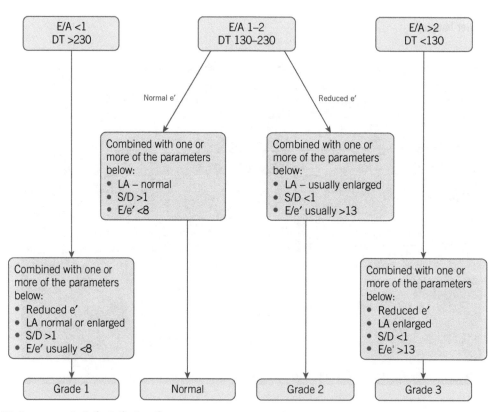

Figure 3.15 Assessment of diastolic function.

pathology, fluid balance, organ support, and drug therapy.

In a steady physiological state, we ask one overall question of diastolic data—how can we characterize diastolic function as a global parameter? By contrast, in critical illness, diastolic assessment answers two separate physiological questions:

1. How well is the myocardium currently relaxing? This is a measure of the energy-requiring diastolic capacity.

2. What is the left ventricular filling pressure at the time of assessment? This is a measure of the moment-to-moment LVEDP.

Practice point

- In critical illness, diastolic assessment requires independent assessment and interpretation of left ventricular relaxation and left ventricular filling pressures, as they are not directly related in this physiological state.

- A diagnosis of diastolic dysfunction should only be assigned 6–8 weeks following resolution of critical illness when diastolic data can be re-assessed in a steady physiological state.

Left ventricular relaxation

Tissue Doppler has been validated as a relatively preload- and afterload-independent measure of left ventricular relaxation, especially when it is measured at the lateral annulus. Normal e' minimum values are 8 cm/s at the septal mitral annulus and 10 cm/s at the lateral mitral annulus, or an average of 9 cm/s. Values below this represent a state of impaired ventricular relaxation.

Left ventricular filling pressures

Doppler studies in patients with right heart catheters have shown that echocardiography can be used to estimate filling pressures in critically unwell patients using the ratio between the E wave as a representative of transmitral passive left ventricular filling and e' as a load-independent marker of left ventricular relaxation. Together these measurements evidence the current LVEDP—the equivalent of a pulmonary capillary wedge pressure. An average E/e' ratio <8 is normal, whereas an average E/e' ratio >13 indicates a raised LVEDP. When patients are in the grey area in between, ancillary measures can be used, as illustrated in Figure 3.16. Echocardiographic estimation of the LVEDP is a vital point of care investigation—it can raise the suspicion of cardiogenic pulmonary oedema in undifferentiated hypoxaemia and can help identify the cause.

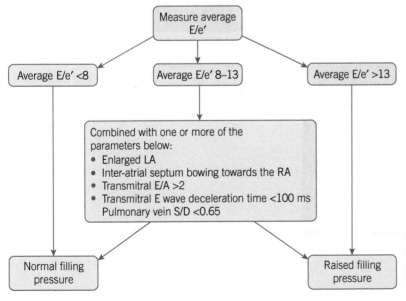

Figure 3.16 Assessment of left ventricular filling pressures in critical illness.

CASE STUDY

A patient on the ICU has persistent hypoxia—would he benefit from diuresis?

A 62-year-old man was admitted to the ICU with severe sepsis secondary to bronchopneumonia. He had a history of hypertension and was a moderate smoker. He was intubated in the emergency department and resuscitated with intravenous fluids and antibiotics. Six days into his ICU stay, his gas exchange remained poor. A bedside chest radiograph was performed (Figure 3.17).

His fluid balance was positive by 6 L (length of stay), and a differential diagnosis was made of non-resolving pneumonia or interstitial oedema. Bedside TTE was performed. It showed normal biventricular structure and function. Aside from mild TR, the heart valves were intact. His left ventricular filling pressure was estimated (Figure 3.18).

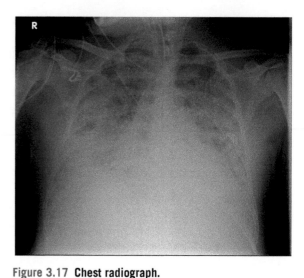

Figure 3.17 Chest radiograph.

© Oxford University Hospitals NHS Foundation Trust 2016, with permission.

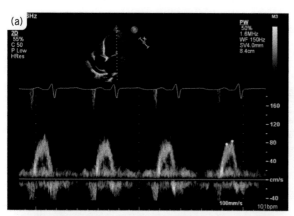

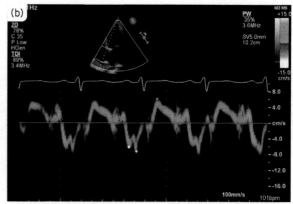

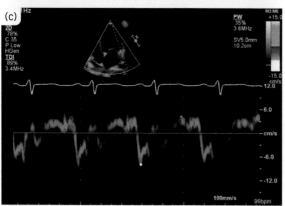

Figure 3.18 (a), (b), and (c) Stills used to estimate left ventricular filling pressure.

© Oxford University Hospitals NHS Foundation Trust 2016, with permission.

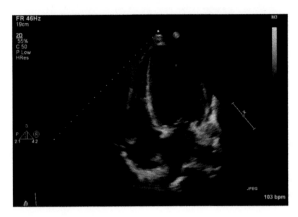

Figure 3.19 Deviation of the inter-atrial septum towards the right atrium.
© Oxford University Hospitals NHS Foundation Trust 2016, with permission.

The E/e′ ratio was 11, so ancillary measures were used. The left atrial volume was measured at 97 mL (severely dilated), and the inter-atrial septum was deviated towards the right atrium (Figure 3.19). A diagnosis of raised LVEDP was made, and he was commenced on a furosemide infusion. His fluid balance for the following 24-hour period was 2.5 L negative, with a marked improvement in gas exchange.

Causes of diastolic dysfunction in critically ill patients

There are two groups of critically ill patients in whom the diastolic phase is relevant to management:

- Those patients with pre-existing diastolic dysfunction
- Those patients in whom we find evidence of impaired left ventricular relaxation without known prior diastolic dysfunction.

Practice point

This second group should not be labelled as having diastolic dysfunction until diastolic data are repeated at 6–8 weeks.

Table 3.1 shows both pre-existing and acute risk factors for impaired left ventricular relaxation during critical illness and helps us to identify vulnerable individuals.

Incidence of diastolic dysfunction in critically ill patients and association with mortality

Heart failure affects 0.6–0.9% of the UK population, and 13% of the male population over the age of 75. Approximately one-third of heart failure patients have a normal or near-normal EF, and significantly diastolic heart failure has a very similar attributable mortality at 1 and 5 years following hospitalization to systolic heart failure.

Recent data from sepsis studies have shown that over two-thirds of patients with septic shock have systolic impairment. The incidence of diastolic dysfunction in sepsis and any association with mortality has been relatively understudied. A recent systematic review identified 19 studies of diastolic function assessed with TDi in critically ill adults with a total of 1365 patients. It found an incidence of diastolic dysfunction of 20–92%. Ten of the studies looked for a mortality association; three of them found that it was an independent predictor of mortality (Table 3.2).

Management of the critically ill patient with diastolic dysfunction

The management of critically ill patients with diastolic dysfunction can be challenging. Impairment of left ventricular relaxation reduces diastolic filling, leading to a reduced SV and a fall in cardiac output. Any compensatory tachycardia can make matters worse, as this will further shorten the diastolic filling time. Additionally, the rise in left atrial pressure that is required to maintain left ventricular filling is reflected in the pulmonary venous system, leading to pulmonary congestion (Figure 3.20).

The physiological sequelae of diastolic dysfunction result in a delicate balance between a preload that is sufficient to maintain cardiac output versus excessive left ventricular filling pressures resulting in pulmonary oedema. The management principles include:

- Avoidance of precipitating factors
- Treatment of any underlying causes
- Treatment of the physiological sequelae

Table 3.1 Risk factors for impaired left ventricular relaxation during critical illness

Pre-existing	Comments
Age	Incidence increases with age
Gender	Increased incidence female:male
Hypertension	Leads to LVH
Diabetes	Leads to LVH and fibrosis
Chronic kidney disease	A multifactorial effect—association with ischaemic heart disease, diabetes, early fibrosis in association with amyloid deposits
Valvular heart disease	Leads to LVH
Ischaemic heart disease	Slows ventricular relaxation and impairs distensibility
Obesity	Associated with diastolic dysfunction independent of cardiovascular risk factors
Myocardial disorders	Examples include hypertrophic cardiomyopathy, infiltrative conditions, and pericardial disease
Acute illness	
Sepsis	Likely related to nitration of contractile proteins, resulting in impaired left ventricular relaxation and reduced left ventricular compliance
Hypoxia/acidosis	Likely related to proteins governing calcium removal from the cytosol during diastole
Acute kidney injury	Metabolic derangement
Myocardial ischaemia	One of the main mechanisms of diastolic dysfunction in the critically ill, secondary to sympathetic activation, shivering, anaemia, hypovolaemia, and hypoxia. Results in impairment of left ventricular relaxation
Therapy	
Mechanical ventilation	Positive pressure ventilation increases intracardiac pressure and inhibits left ventricular filling PEEP reduces left ventricular compliance
Sedatives	Propofol and ketamine are associated with impaired left ventricular relaxation and reduced left ventricular compliance
Inotropes/vasopressors	• Adrenaline enhances left ventricular relaxation • Noradrenaline impairs left ventricular relaxation • Dobutamine, enoximone, and levosimendan improve left ventricular relaxation and compliance
Withdrawal of medications	Beta blockers (lead to tachycardia and reduced diastolic filling time)
Physiology	
Haemodynamic changes	Sympathetic tone, preload, afterload
Extrinsic compression of the cardiac chambers	Abdominal hypertension, pleural effusions, pericardial effusions, high levels of PEEP

Table 3.2 Association of diastolic dysfunction with mortality

Subgroup of patients in study	Number of patients	Mortality
General ICU patients	58	• Patients with diastolic dysfunction had a reduced in-hospital survival (37% vs 83%, $p = 0.001$) • Diastolic dysfunction was a significant univariate predictor of in-hospital mortality by Cox regression analysis
General ICU patients	94	• No difference in diastolic function (survivors vs non-survivors at 28 days) $e' = 8.7 \pm 2.7$ cm/s vs 9.1 ± 3.5 cm/s, $p = 0.58$
SIRS and shock	49	• No difference in diastolic function (survivors vs non-survivors at 1 year) Median $e' = 8.4$ (7.5–10.8) vs 7.9 (6.3–9.6), non-significant
Septic shock	35	• No difference in diastolic function (survivors vs non-survivors at hospital discharge) $e' = 11.4$ (9.1–16.0) vs 12 (11.1–13.4)
Severe sepsis or septic shock	45	• Difference in diastolic function (survivors vs non-survivors at hospital discharge) $E' = 13.2 \pm 4.7$ vs 10.1 ± 3.7 ($p = 0.03$)
Severe sepsis or septic shock	262	• Difference in diastolic function (survivors vs non-survivors at 2-year follow-up) Septal $e' = 9.3 \pm 3.4$ vs 6.8 ± 2.2 cm/s ($p < 0.0001$) Lateral $e' = 11.3 \pm 4.1$ vs 9.0 ± 3.5 cm/s ($p < 0.0001$) • Cox multivariate survival analysis showed reduced septal e' was the strongest independent predictor of mortality (at hospital discharge)
Severe sepsis or septic shock	106	• Difference in diastolic function (survivors vs non-survivors at hospital discharge) Septal $e' = 8.6 \pm 2.8$ vs 7.5 ± 2.2 cm/s ($p = 0.038$) Lateral $e' = 12.5 \pm 3.3$ vs 10.4 ± 3.2 cm/s ($p = 0.004$)
Severe sepsis or septic shock	106	• No survival difference between group with diastolic dysfunction and normal myocardium group 30-day mortality = 15 (38%) vs 16 (42%); $p = 0.74$ 1-year mortality = 26 (67%) vs 21 (55%); $p = 0.30$
Cancer and septic shock	45	• Difference in the incidence of diastolic dysfunction (survivors vs non-survivors on the ICU) 6 (26%) vs 12 (54.5%); $p = 0.07$
Cancer and septic shock	72	• Difference in diastolic function (survivors vs non-survivors on the ICU) $e' <8$ 8 (21.3%) vs 25 (71.4%); $p < 0.001$ • $e' <8$ independently associated with ICU mortality (OR 7.7, 95% CI 2.58–23.38; $p < 0.001$)

CI, confidence interval; ICU, intensive care unit; OR, odds ratio; SIRS, systemic inflammatory response syndrome.

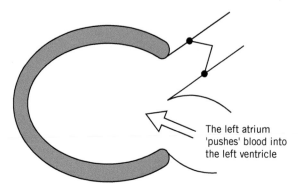

The left atrium 'pushes' blood into the left ventricle

Figure 3.20 A rise in left atrial pressure is needed to maintain left ventricular filling when left ventricular relaxation is impaired.

- Any acute illnesses or physiological derangements that are associated with diastolic dysfunction should be identified and treated (for example, hypoxia, myocardial ischaemia, hypertension, and tachyarrhythmias)

- Rationalizing ICU therapies that are associated with diastolic dysfunction such as mechanical ventilation and vasopressors

- Cautious use of fluids. Fluid overload can be treated with vasodilators, diuretics, or renal replacement therapy, whereas raised left ventricular filling pressures can be treated with NIV. There is no current therapy that specifically treats left ventricular diastolic dysfunction.

CASE STUDY

The patient on the ICU with impaired left ventricular relaxation

A 76-year-old patient was admitted to the ICU post-emergency laparotomy for faecal peritonitis. She had a history of hypertension and ischaemic heart disease. She was treated for Gram-negative sepsis and after 6 days was successfully weaned from mechanical ventilation and respiratory support. She achieved her nutritional targets via enteral feeding and mobilized successfully with the physiotherapy team. Discharge planning was initiated, but on day 9 she became acutely short of breath, and the attending doctor was called to the bedspace as 'she needed intubation'. The patient was in sinus rhythm with a pulse of 128, a blood pressure of 196/112, and a respiratory rate of 32. Saturations were maintained at 98% with a waters circuit. Rapid bedside examination did not reveal any new significant clinical signs, and a differential diagnosis was made of pulmonary embolism (PE) or a cardiac event. A bedside TTE was performed. It showed normal left ventricular systolic function with moderate concentric LVH, a normal right heart, and normal valves and pericardium. Doppler echocardiography revealed a raised LVEDP (Figure 3.21).

A diagnosis of hypertensive pulmonary oedema was made in a patient with a stiff LV secondary to LVH. The patient was treated with an intravenous vasodilator, intravenous morphine, and PEEP via the waters circuit. Over the next 15 min, the patient was weaned successfully onto low-flow face mask oxygen. A review of her drug chart revealed an omission of her usual antihypertensive medication. This was restarted, and she was discharged uneventfully the following day.

Diastolic function and weaning from mechanical ventilation

Failed extubation is defined as reintubation within 48–72 hours after planned extubation from mechanical ventilation. A decision to extubate is carefully considered since reintubation is associated with increased duration of hospital stay, significant morbidity such as pneumonia, and mortality. The median reintubation rate is approximately 15% in current UK practice.

Factors affecting a decision to extubate include:

- Current level of respiratory support

- Resolution of underlying pathology

- Neurological status

- Response to a spontaneous breathing trial (SBT)— where the loading conditions of spontaneous unassisted respiration are simulated.

Clinicians are careful to observe the patient's cardiovascular response to an SBT, looking for features predictive of weaning failure such as tachycardia, hyper- or hypotension, and pulmonary oedema. The

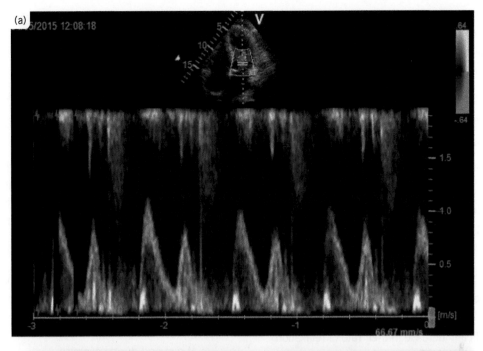

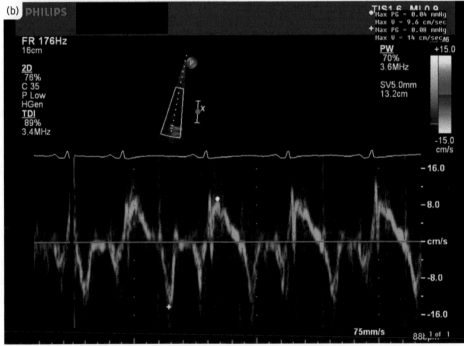

Figure 3.21 Doppler echocardiography consistent with a raised LVEDP.

© Oxford University Hospitals NHS Foundation Trust 2016, with permission.

increased effort of breathing during weaning from a ventilator is akin to physical exercise.

Withdrawal of positive pressure ventilation causes the following cardiovascular impact:

- Increased venous return
- Increased left ventricular afterload
- Decreased left ventricular compliance
- A propensity to coronary ischaemia.

Failure of weaning due to cardiovascular impact can be predicted by looking at left ventricular compliance and filling pressures prior to, and during, a trial of spontaneous breathing.

- Patients who wean successfully have a:
  - Higher rate of left ventricular relaxation (e') on their baseline TTE
  - Significant increase in their rate of relaxation during their SBT
- Left ventricular filling pressures are lower at baseline and during a breathing trial in those who wean successfully
- Left ventricular filling pressures rise, usually from a higher starting point in those who fail to wean
- There is an 80% prevalence of impaired left ventricular relaxation in those who fail to wean
- This effect is seen even in the absence of left ventricular systolic dysfunction.

Practice point

Evidence suggests that an E/e' ratio measured 10 min into an SBT of >14.5 predicts weaning failure with a sensitivity of 75% and a specificity of 95.8%.

Multiple choice questions

1. The assessment of diastolic function:
   A Is made using quantitative data only
   B Is the same in health and in critical illness
   C Is a useful measure of fluid responsiveness
   D In critical illness represents the diastolic function in health

   E Can help predict failure to wean from mechanical ventilation

2. When assessing diastolic function:
   A e' is relatively load-independent
   B The E/e' ratio can be used to estimate left ventricular filling pressures in health
   C The E/e' ratio can be used to estimate left ventricular filling pressures in critically ill patients
   D Ventricular relaxation and left ventricular filling pressures are directly related in health
   E Ventricular relaxation and left ventricular filling pressures are directly related in critical illness

3. Regarding diastole:
   A It is an entirely passive process
   B It is divided into two physiological phases
   C Atrial contraction accounts for approximately 10–20% of left ventricular filling
   D In health, the left atrial pressure is normal, both at rest and during exercise
   E Left ventricular filling occurs during the first phase

4. Regarding diastolic dysfunction:
   A All patients with diastolic dysfunction also have a degree of systolic dysfunction
   B Diastolic dysfunction is an abnormality of left ventricular distensibility, filling, or relaxation
   C As the left ventricle becomes stiffer, a higher left atrial pressure is needed to maintain filling
   D Patients with diastolic dysfunction tolerate atrial fibrillation well
   E Certain therapies used in critical illness can worsen diastolic function

5. Regarding diastolic dysfunction:
   A Myocardial ischaemia is a common cause of diastolic dysfunction in the critically ill
   B An ageing population with an increasing comorbid load means that more patients with preexisting diastolic dysfunction are being admitted to the intensive care unit
   C Assessment of diastolic function during critical illness may not be representative of the patient's baseline cardiac function
   D Dobutamine may play a role in enhancing left ventricular relaxation
   E Doppler measures should be obtained at end-inspiration

For answers to multiple choice questions, please see 'Appendix 1: Answers to multiple choice questions', p. 171.

Further reading

Aurigemma GP, Gaasch WH. Clinical practice. Diastolic heart failure. *N Engl J Med* 2004; **351**: 1097–105.

Jacques DC, Pinsky MR, Severyn D, Gorcsan J 3rd. Influence of alterations in loading on mitral annular velocity by tissue Doppler echocardiography and its associated ability to predict filling pressures. *Chest* 2004; **126**: 1910–18.

Moschietto S, Doyen D, Grech L, Dellamonica J, Hyvernat H, Bernardin G. Transthoracic echocardiography with Doppler tissue imaging predicts weaning failure from mechanical ventilation: evolution of the left ventricle relaxation rate during a spontaneous breathing trial is the key factor in weaning outcome. *Crit Care* 2012; **16**: R81.

Nagueh SF, Appleton CP, Gillebert TC, *et al.* Recommendations for the evaluation of left ventricular diastolic function by echocardiography. *Eur J Echocardiogr* 2009; **10**: 165–93.

Vignon P, Allot V, Lesage J, *et al*. Diagnosis of left ventricular diastolic dysfunction in the setting of acute changes in loading conditions. *Crit Care* 2007; **11**: R43.

4

The right ventricle in critical illness

The right heart

The right ventricle plays an important role in maintaining cardiac output in physiology and pathophysiology. Early understanding of the right heart regarded it as a conduit for passage of blood from the caval veins to the pulmonary circulation. It has not been till the last few decades that the importance of the right ventricle as a contractile pump has emerged.

The heart is a circuit in series, and the lungs are the only organs to receive the entire cardiac output. Although the two sides of the heart move the same volume of blood, they generate their cardiac output very differently. The RV is anatomically very different from the LV, and so the parameters used to assess its performance must be different too.

Right heart structure and function

The right atrium receives the complete systemic venous return from the superior and inferior venae cavae, which then passes through the tricuspid valve to the RV, following ejection of blood in the main pulmonary trunk.

The pulmonary vasculature displays some unique and physiologically important anatomical features.

* The pulmonary arteries are large in calibre and thin-walled.

* The pulmonary vascular bed has a large reserve for recruitment of vascular segments that are normally not perfused.

* The pulmonary circulation is a low-pressure, high-capacitance system capable of large increases in

blood flow, but resulting in only minimal increases in pressure.

The RV itself is a thin-walled structure, which acts as a capacitance reservoir and responds poorly to acute increases in afterload. The two ventricles are in series but interact since they lie next to each other within the pericardial sac. The compliance of one can therefore directly affect the other.

The RV is in continuity with the rest of the heart but has an entirely separate embryological origin. The RV and outflow tract are developed from the anterior heart field. The right atrium and left-sided chambers are derived from the primary heart field.

The RV has a distinct genetic and neurohormonal make-up from the rest of the heart. With increasing afterload, the right ventricular response profile in messenger ribonucleic acid (mRNA) and protein expression is different to the LV.

Macroscopically, the RV at the apex has a triangular cross-section. Moving towards the base of the heart, it has a crescenteric shape. The RV is made up of an inflow area, a trabeculated apex, and a smooth outflow or infundibulum leading into the PA. The heavy trabeculations allow the RV to acutely dilate to accommodate increases in volume. The RV and PA act as, and should be regarded as, a coupled unit.

The muscle fibres of the RV are arranged in two sets—the inner longitudinal fibres and the subepicardial circumferential fibres that are in continuity with the LV. This means that the longitudinal fibres provide a greater contribution to contractility than for the LV, generating a bellows effect from the apex to the base. Contraction of the LV also contributes to some of the stroke work of the RV through the interconnection of the subepicardial fibres. The RV has one-sixth of the muscle mass of the LV and performs one-quarter of the left ventricular stroke work.

Right ventricular contraction occurs in a sequential manner, starting first at the apex and ending at the infundibulum. This results in a peristaltic type of contraction.

Key features of right ventricular peristaltic movement are:

- Infundibular expansion occurs just prior to contraction
- Infundibular contraction occurs 20–50 ms after contraction of the right ventricular free wall
- Longitudinal shortening contributes most to right ventricular free wall contraction
- The right ventricular free wall also moves in towards the left ventricular septum, referred to as transverse shortening
- The LV contributes to right ventricular ejection by bulging into the right ventricular cavity and pressuring the blood
- Low pressure within the pulmonary vasculature encourages blood flow to continue forwards, even after the right ventricular pressure has decreased to a value below that of the PA.

The two pressure–volume loops (Figure 4.1) demonstrate the differences between the left and right systems.

- The left ventricular loop is rectangular in shape, reflecting an acute rise in pressure with left ventricular filling, whereas that of the RV is more triangular.
- During right ventricular filling, right ventricular volume increases with very little increase in pressure.
- The right ventricular isovolaemic contraction phase is of short duration due to low pressure in the PA.

The RV is relatively well protected against ischaemia since oxygen requirements are less due to low preload and afterload. Due to the lower wall tension generated by the RV, blood flow within the coronary arteries supplying the right heart occurs both in diastole and systole. The right ventricular free wall is also supplied dually by the right coronary and left coronary arteries. Due to these factors, under stress, the RV is able to increase its oxygen extraction. The caveat to this is

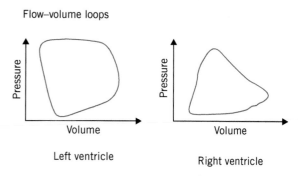

Figure 4.1 **Left and right ventricle pressure–volume loops.**

that an acute rise in left ventricular wall tension can dramatically reduce right coronary blood flow.

Right ventricle–pulmonary artery coupling

Figure 4.2 demonstrates the pressures normally generated by the right heart within the RV–PA system.
The RV is a low-pressure, high-capacitance system which pumps the entire cardiac output into a low-resistance, highly compliant vascular bed. In the normal individual, the RV only needs to generate systolic pressures of 25 mmHg, compared to 120 mmHg in the LV. The compliance of the pulmonary system is 2 mL/mmHg.

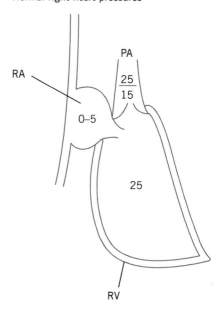

Figure 4.2 **Normal right heart pressures.**

Therefore, by extrapolation, we can conclude that:

- The RV tolerates PA pressure changes poorly
- The RV can accommodate and react appropriately to changes in volume.

Due to the unique anatomy and physiology of the RV, we should only view the RV as a coupled unit with the PA and never in isolation.

Changes in PA tension are directly reflected in the:

- Acute dysfunction or
- Chronic adaptation of the RV.

> **Practice point**
>
> In order to understand the behaviour of the RV, the RV and PA must be viewed as a coupled unit—this is known as RV–PA coupling.

Understanding the effects of an acute or chronic rise in pulmonary vascular resistance

Acute cor pulmonale refers to acute right ventricular failure in the setting of acutely elevated pulmonary vascular resistance (PVR) due to an acute disease process affecting the lungs. PHT is frequently encountered on the ICU secondary to:

- Pneumonia or pneumonitis
- Acute PE
- Adult respiratory distress syndrome and hypoxaemic vasoconstriction
- Overventilation.

The pressure in the pulmonary system depends on cardiac output, resistance, and compliance. It is common to see a minor rise in pulmonary arterial pressure due to a rise in cardiac output, but it is important to detect a significant increase in pulmonary arterial hypertension since this is an independent predictor of mortality in the conditions listed above.

Our current focus in the critically ill ventilated patient is on prevention of further pulmonary damage. However, our new understanding of the impact of ventilation and underlying pulmonary pathology on the right heart is beginning to shift this focus back to looking at the heart and lungs as a unit. The aim of 'protective ventilation' should be to reduce further pulmonary damage and maintain right heart function.

Without time to hypertrophy and accommodate a rise in pulmonary artery pressure (PAP), the RV is unable to tolerate a pressure increase of >40 mmHg mean PAP. At this pressure level, RV failure will ensue. Therefore, when the heart has previously been normal in structure and function, a sudden rise in PVR and PAP will be reflected by a rise in measured pressures, but more significantly by evidence of **failure of the RV**.

Conversely, where the right heart has been subjected to a prolonged period of rising PVR and PAP, the RV will hypertrophy to maintain RV–PA coupling and therefore generate higher PAP than we see in the acute setting.

These two key physiological situations are shown in Figure 4.3 demonstrating the anatomical and pressure changes seen in acute and chronic right heart strain.

> **Practice point**
>
> The response of the RV to a rise in PVR is determined by chronicity:
>
> - An acute rise in pressure will cause the RV to fail: right ventricular structural and functional assessment is therefore crucial.
> - A chronic rise in pressure will cause the RV to hypertrophy: right ventricular structural and functional assessment is therefore crucial.

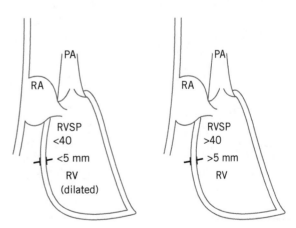

Figure 4.3 The left image shows the changes associated with acute right heart strain, and the right image with chronic right heart strain.

Assessing pulmonary artery pressures and pulmonary vascular resistance

PAP and PVR are not synonymous. Although pulmonary artery systolic pressure (PASP) and PVR usually vary synchronously in critically ill patients, an elevation in PASP does not always imply an increase in PVR. The relationship Δ pressure = flow × resistance reminds us that an increase in pressure can be due to an increase in either cardiac output or PVR. To calculate a non-invasive index of PVR, the ratio of the peak tricuspid regurgitant velocity to the velocity time integral in the right ventricular outflow tract (RVOT) can be used. The normal ratio is ≤0.15.

Figure 4.4 shows this calculation in action.

Measuring pulmonary artery systolic pressure

PASP can be estimated by the assessment of a TR velocity (TRV) jet. Recent cohort studies have demonstrated that a TR jet can be found in almost 100% of subjects. Using a continuous-wave Doppler trace, the tricuspid valve pressure gradient can be calculated from the modified Bernoulli equation, as shown below; when added to the right atrial pressure (RAP), an estimate of the RVSP is obtained.

$$RVSP = 4 \times TRV^2 + RAP \, mmHg$$

In the absence of a gradient across the pulmonary valve or RVOT, the PASP is equal to the RVSP. Velocity measurements are angle-dependent, so it is recommended that multiple views are taken to gain TR signals in several windows and to use the signal with the highest velocity. An optimal trace and measurement are shown in Figure 4.5.

Normal resting values are defined as a peak TR gradient of ≤2.8 m/s or a peak systolic pressure of 35 mmHg. This value may increase with age or increasing body surface area (BSA). In patients with severe TR, there is early equalization of right ventricular and right atrial pressures, so the Doppler envelope becomes unclear, as shown in Figure 4.6, and use of the simplified Bernoulli equation may underestimate the true pressure gradient.

The RAP is estimated by assessing the size and respirophasic changes of the IVC. The IVC should be assessed in the subcostal view. The diameter of the IVC should be measured perpendicular to its long axis at end-expiration, just proximal to the junction of the hepatic veins. The hepatic veins usually lie within 0.5–3 cm proximal to the ostium of the RA. See Table 4.1 for guidelines from the American Society of Echocardiography on the assessment of the RAP.

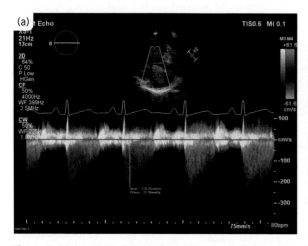
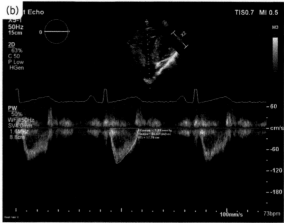

Figure 4.4 (a) and (b) **Calculation of the non-invasive index of pulmonary vascular resistance (PVR).** The ratio of the peak tricuspid regurgitant velocity (2.23 m/s) to the velocity time integral (VTI) in the right ventricular outflow tract (RVOT) (17 cm) is normal at 0.13 (normal <0.15).

© Oxford University Hospitals NHS Foundation Trust 2016, with permission.

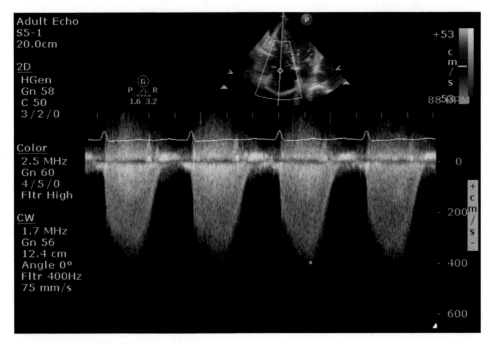

Figure 4.5 Tricuspid regurgitation Doppler trace.
© Oxford University Hospitals NHS Foundation Trust 2016, with permission.

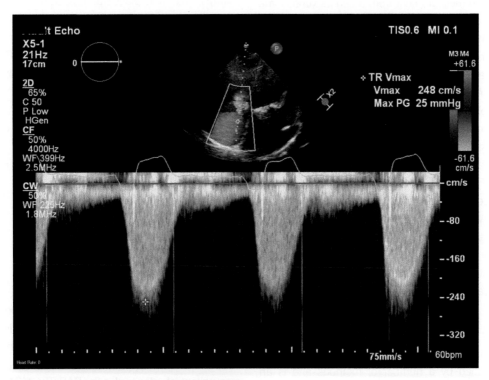

Figure 4.6 Doppler envelope in severe tricuspid regurgitation.
© Oxford University Hospitals NHS Foundation Trust 2016, with permission.

Table 4.1 Guidelines for assessment of RAP

IVC collapse with Sniff	IVC diameter	
	≤2.1 cm	≥2.1 cm
Yes	Normal RAP (0–5 mmHg)	Intermediate RAP (5–10 mmHg)
No	Intermediate RAP (5–10 mmHg)	High RAP (15 mmHg)

Adapted from *Journal of the American Society of Echocardiography*, 23, Rudski, L.G., Wyman W. L., Afilalo, J. et al., 'Guidelines for the Echocardiographic Assessment of the Right Heart in Adults: A Report from the American Society of Echocardiography', pp. 685–713, Copyright 2010, with permission from the American Society of Echocardiography.

These parameters work well when assessing the low or high values of RAP, but less so when assessing intermediate values. In patients ventilated with mechanical ventilation, the degree of IVC collapse cannot be reliably used to estimate the RAP since the IVC is increasingly splinted with increasingly mandatory modes ventilation. The pressure measurement from a central venous line should then be used, if present. In ventilated patients, an IVC diameter of <12 mm appears accurate in identifying patients with RAPs <10 mmHg.

Secondary indices of RAP estimation can also be used. At low or normal RAP, there is predominantly systolic flow in the hepatic veins. As RAP rises, there is a reversal, so the velocity of the diastolic flow becomes greater than the velocity of the systolic flow. These changes have been validated in ventilated patients. Figure 4.7 gives an example of abnormal diastolic dominance in the hepatic veins.

A qualitative inspection of the inter-atrial septum can also be used as a surrogate measurement of RAP. When the inter-atrial septum bulges towards the LA throughout the cardiac cycle, then this is consistent with a raised RAP of >15 mmHg.

Measuring mean pulmonary artery pressure

The mean pulmonary artery pressure (MPAP) can be determined by a number of methods and is an important component of looking for pulmonary arterial hypertension, since studies of the accuracy of Doppler techniques for the assessment of PAP show the strongest correlation with right heart catheter data when the mean pressure is measured using Doppler. The MPAP can be calculated in the same way as mean arterial pressure by using the equation:

$$MPAP = 1/3(PASP) + 2/3(PADP)$$

The MPAP can be derived from the PASP by using the equation:

$$MPAP = 0.6 \times PASP + 2\,mmHg$$

Pulmonary acceleration time

Another way to estimate the MPAP is to look at the time from the beginning of flow to peak flow of blood at the RVOT. This is termed the pulmonary acceleration time (AT). As the PAP rises, the AT decreases, provided the heart rate is normal (60–100 bpm). The normal value is >110 ms, and the abnormal value is anything <105 ms.

The AT is measured from the onset of flow to the onset of peak pulmonary flow velocity. The Doppler sample volume is placed at the centre of the pulmonary artery in the short axis view, as shown Figure 4.8. This measurement is affected by the heart rate and should be corrected if the heart rate is >100 bpm or <70 bpm; heart rate correction is achieved by multiplying by 75 and dividing by the heart rate. The Doppler envelope can also be assessed qualitatively; if there is notching of the envelope, this is suggestive of a rise of the PVR, as shown in Figure 4.9.

The MPAP can also be estimated using the equation:

$$MPAP = 79 - (0.45 \times AT)$$

$$MPAP = 90 - (0.62 \times AT) \text{ if } AT < 120\,ms$$

Pulmonary regurgitant jet

Where a pulmonary regurgitant jet can be clearly seen, then the MPAP is equal to the pressure gradient calculated from the peak velocity plus the RAP. The DPAP is equal to the pressure gradient calculated from the end regurgitant jet velocity plus the RAP. The MPAP can also be calculated from the mean systolic pressure produced from the TR jet velocity time integral plus the RAP.

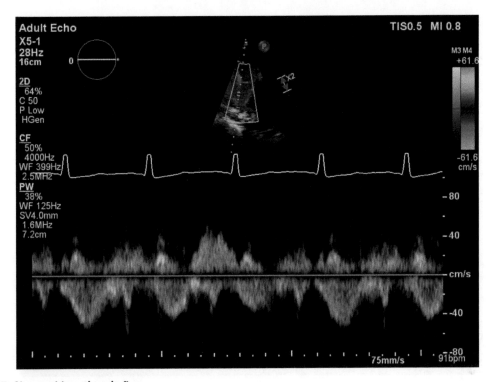

Figure 4.7 Abnormal hepatic vein flow.
© Oxford University Hospitals NHS Foundation Trust 2016, with permission.

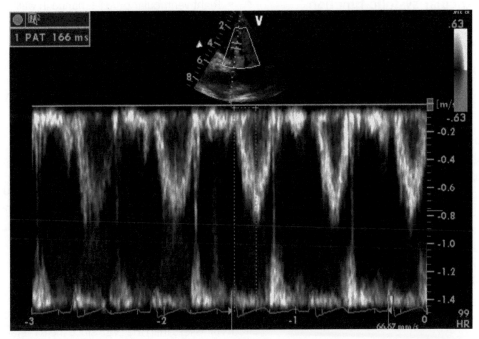

Figure 4.8 Position of pulsed-wave Doppler across the pulmonary valve to assess the acceleration time.
© Oxford University Hospitals NHS Foundation Trust 2016, with permission.

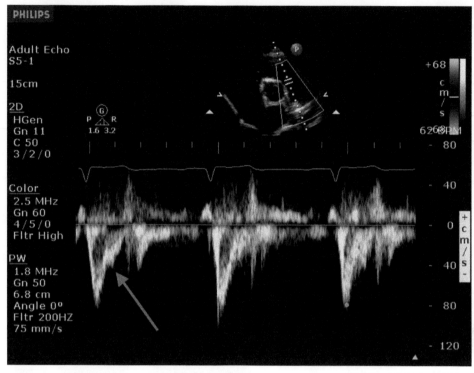

Figure 4.9 Notching of the pulmonary artery Doppler envelope.
© Oxford University Hospitals NHS Foundation Trust 2016, with permission.

Right ventricular systolic function

Practice point

Even though it is important to consider PAP and PVR, in the acute setting, the most important feature of the RV is its function.

When assessing the function of the RV, we need to be mindful of the dominance of longitudinal contraction in right ventricular function. In contrast, the LV relies mainly upon radial contraction, and function is therefore assessable from multiple cross-sectional views. An ideal index of contractility should be independent of loading conditions and ventricular size but sensitive to changes in inotropy.

Right ventricular systolic function should ideally be assessed by a number of indices.

Global assessment methods of right ventricular function include:

- Right ventricular ejection fraction (RVEF)

- Right ventricular dP/dT (change in wall pressure/ time)

- FAC

- Myocardial performance index (MPI).

Regional assessment methods of right ventricular function include:

- TAPSE

- TDi of the tricuspid annulus systolic velocity.

Qualitative assessment of right ventricular function by careful inspection is also an important component of assessment of the RV and a useful correlate where a regional method is used alone.

Right ventricular ejection fraction

RVEF is a load-dependent marker of function. The RVEF is less than the LVEF since the RV retains a larger volume during diastole. RVEF has a quoted normal range of 40–76%, validated by MRI, which can view the RV in three dimensions. The RV and outflow tract have a bellows and spout structure, which is difficult to model accurately from 2D to 3D imaging. Therefore, performing RVEF measurement using 2D echocardiography is less accurate than 3D imaging modalities and has a correlation of 0.65–0.8, when compared to MRI or radionuclide angiography.

Right ventricular dP/dT

Right ventricular dP/dT is a measure of the rate of pressure rise in the RV over a fixed time period and is an index of ventricular contractility. It is more often used for assessment of the LV and relies upon the presence of a MR jet. Figure 4.10 demonstrates how dP/dT is measured using MR on the left side of the heart.

For right ventricular assessment, continuous-wave Doppler is placed across the tricuspid valve annulus. If a complete tricuspid regurgitation envelope is achieved, the time required for the tricuspid

regurgitation jet to increase in velocity from 1 to 2 m/s is measured, as shown for the mitral valve above. According to the modified Bernoulli equation, this represents a 12 mmHg increase in pressure (4 mmHg to 16 mmHg). The dP/dT is calculated by dividing 12 mmHg by the time measured in seconds. However, this remains a load-dependent variable, and there are limited normal range data for this measurement.

Right ventricular fractional area change

In contrast to the measurement of RVEF using the Simpson's biplane method, no geometric assumptions are made in the measurement of right ventricular fractional area change (RVFAC), although both measurements are load-dependent. The RVFAC is measured in the 2D apical four-chamber view, according to the equation:

$$\frac{(End\text{-}diastolic\,area)-(End\text{-}systolic\,area)}{(End\text{-}diastolic\,area)}\times100$$

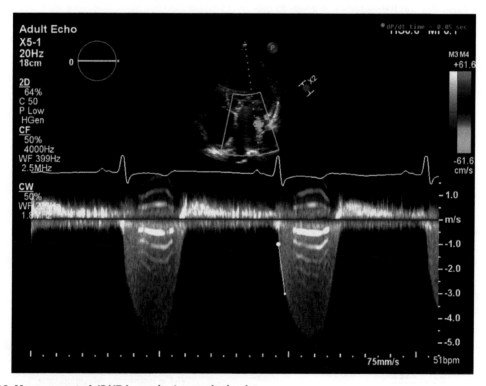

Figure 4.10 Measurement of dP/dT from mitral regurgitation jet.
© Oxford University Hospitals NHS Foundation Trust 2016, with permission.

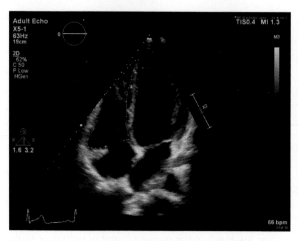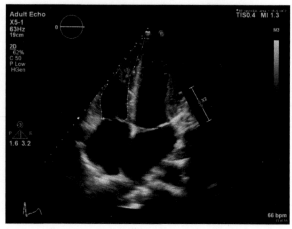

Figure 4.11 The image on the left shows the right ventricular diastolic area and on the right the right ventricular systolic area.

© Oxford University Hospitals NHS Foundation Trust 2016, with permission.

The lower reference range is 35%, and the RVFAC is an independent predictor of mortality and morbidity in studies of PE and MI. The RVFAC correlates well with invasively measured RVEF. Inaccuracies can occur due to problems with incomplete visualization of the right ventricular cavity and endocardial definition. Figure 4.11 illustrates the measurements taken to calculate the RVFAC.

Myocardial performance index

The MPI is a more complex and less often used marker of right ventricular systolic and diastolic function. It is calculated as the ratio between the time taken for the ejection and non-ejection work of the ventricle, according to the following calculation:

$$\left(\begin{array}{c} \text{Isovolaemic relaxation time} \\ + \text{Isovolaemic contraction time} \end{array} \right) / (\text{Ejection time})$$

Usefully, this measure remains valid over a range of heart rates but is unreliable when the RAP is raised or the patient is in an irregular heart rhythm.

The MPI is measured using pulsed-wave Doppler positioned in the right ventricular inflow and outflow tracts, positioned as shown in Figure 4.12.

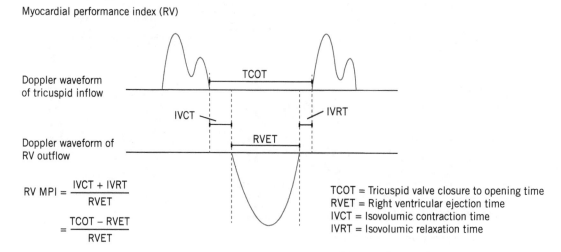

Myocardial performance index (RV)

Doppler waveform of tricuspid inflow

TCOT

IVCT

IVRT

Doppler waveform of RV outflow

RVET

$$\text{RV MPI} = \frac{\text{IVCT} + \text{IVRT}}{\text{RVET}}$$

$$= \frac{\text{TCOT} - \text{RVET}}{\text{RVET}}$$

TCOT = Tricuspid valve closure to opening time
RVET = Right ventricular ejection time
IVCT = Isovolumic contraction time
IVRT = Isovolumic relaxation time

Figure 4.12 Calculation of right ventricular myocardial performance index by pulsed Doppler.

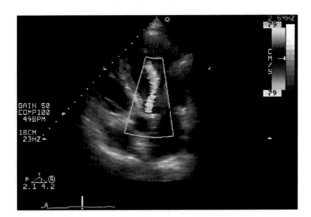

Figure 5.11 [Video 5.5] Apical five-chamber view with a colour Doppler box over the aortic valve and left ventricular outflow tract, demonstrating central aortic regurgitation into the left ventricle.

🔵 *This video is available to watch in the online video appendix.*

© Oxford University Hospitals NHS Foundation Trust 2016, with permission.

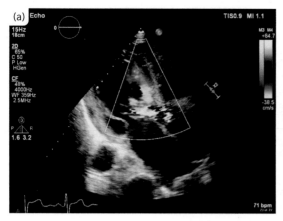 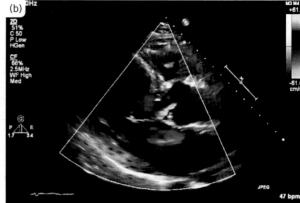

Figure 5.12 (a) [Video 5.6] and 5.12 (b) [Video 5.7] Parasternal long axis view with colour Doppler over the left ventricular outflow tract, demonstrating aortic regurgitation.

🔘 *These videos are available to watch in the online video appendix.*

© Oxford University Hospitals NHS Foundation Trust 2016, with permission.

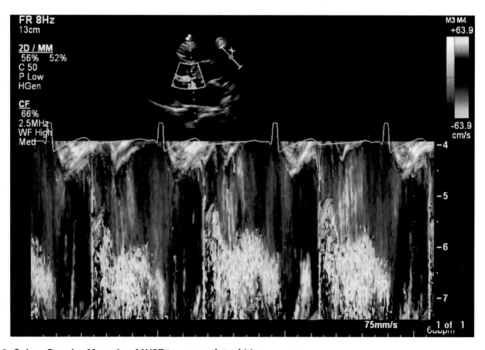

Figure 5.13 Colour Doppler M-mode of LVOT to assess jet width.

© Oxford University Hospitals NHS Foundation Trust 2016, with permission.

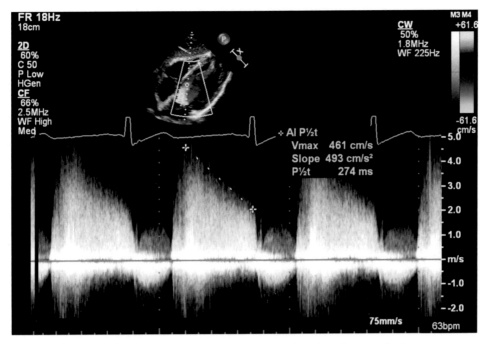

Figure 5.14 **Pressure half-time measurement of continuous-wave Doppler of aortic regurgitation.**

© Oxford University Hospitals NHS Foundation Trust 2016, with permission.

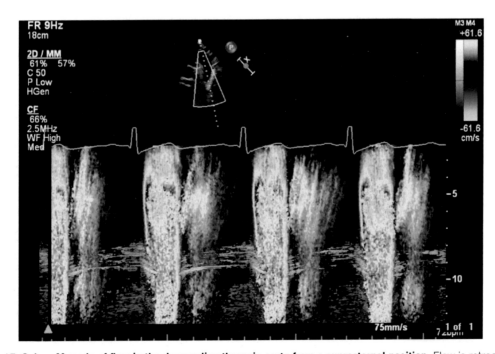

Figure 5.15 **Colour M-mode of flow in the descending thoracic aorta from a suprasternal position.** Flow is retrograde (red) for the whole of diastole due to severe AR.

© Oxford University Hospitals NHS Foundation Trust 2016, with permission.

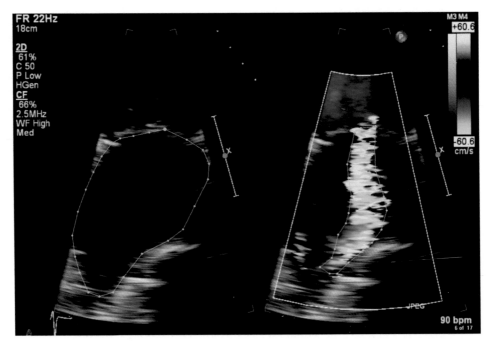

Figure 5.18 [Video 5.9] Estimation of mitral regurgitation jet size, compared to left atrial size from the apical four-chamber position.

⊙ *This video is available to watch in the online video appendix.*

© Oxford University Hospitals NHS Foundation Trust 2016, with permission.

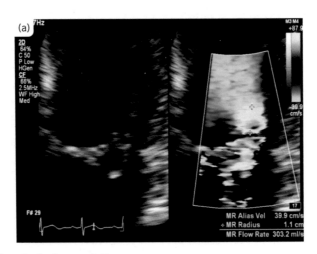

Figure 5.19 (a) Quantification of mitral regurgitation.

© Oxford University Hospitals NHS Foundation Trust 2016, with permission.

This measurement involves two separate images, so care must be taken to ensure the heart rate is reasonably consistent between the two images. An alternative to using the pulsed-wave Doppler technique is to use tissue Doppler. All the time intervals can be measured from one image using tissue Doppler at the tricuspid annulus. The upper limit is 0.40 using the pulsed Doppler method, and 0.55 using the tissue Doppler.

Tricuspid annular plane systolic excursion

This is a very commonly used and useful measure of the longitudinal function of the right ventricular free wall; although this is a regional wall motion assessment, it combines with visual assessment to give a useful, reproducible, and heart rate-independent marker of right ventricular systolic function. There is strong correlation with radionuclide angiography and RVFAC. A decreased TAPSE has also been shown to be independently associated with decreased survival in left heart failure and those with PHT.

The TAPSE is measured using the M-mode, with the cursor placed over the lateral tricuspid annulus in the apical four-chamber view, as shown in Figure 4.13. The degree of longitudinal movement of the annulus is measured as the deepest to the highest movement along one single line of movement. Normal systolic function is >1.6 cm annular plane excursion.

Tissue Doppler imaging

TDi measurement of the longitudinal velocity of the right ventricular contraction is another linear method of assessing right ventricular systolic function. Pulsed-wave Doppler is used to assess the systolic velocity of the RV at the level of the tricuspid annulus. The highest systolic velocity is measured and termed S'. From a number of population studies, the normal cut-off value of >10 cm/s is used. The right ventricular maximum systolic velocity with TDi correlates well with TAPSE and RVFAC. Figure 4.14 demonstrates how TDi is achieved.

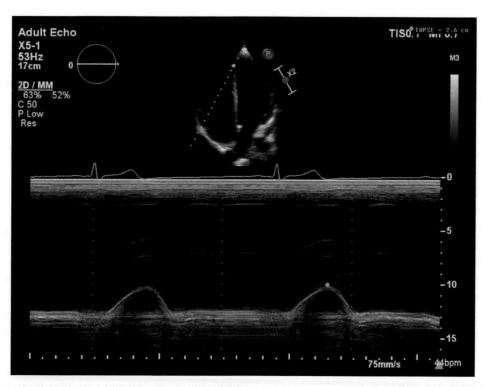

Figure 4.13 Tricuspid annular plane systolic excursion (TAPSE).

© Oxford University Hospitals NHS Foundation Trust 2016, with permission.

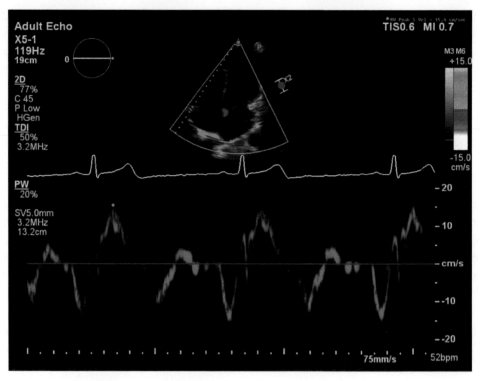

Figure 4.14 Tissue Doppler imaging of the right ventricle.
© Oxford University Hospitals NHS Foundation Trust 2016, with permission.

Right ventricular diastolic function

Right ventricular diastole is composed of many phases, so assessment by one parameter is difficult. It may be an early sign of right ventricular impairment in those with suspected right ventricular impairment or a poor prognostic sign in those with known dysfunction. It is an independent predictor of mortality in chronic heart failure and PHT. Improvement in filling patterns reflects a response to therapy. It could be useful clinically as it can serve as an early marker of subclinical right ventricular dysfunction. Multiple studies have shown that right ventricular diastolic function is usually present before systolic dysfunction or right ventricular dilatation or hypertrophy.

Measurement involves measuring the tricuspid inflow velocities by aligning the Doppler beam at the tricuspid valve and placing the sample volume at the tips of the valve. TDi is used to assess the velocity of the tricuspid annulus. The size of the RA should also be measured. This is measured in end-systole in the apical four-chamber view, and the upper limit of normal is 18 cm².

Grading of diastolic function is as follows:

• Tricuspid E/A ratio <0.8 suggests impaired relaxation

• Tricuspid E/A ratio of 0.8–2.1 with an E/E' >6 suggests pseudonormal filling

• Tricuspid E/A ratio of >2.1 with a deceleration time of <120 ms suggests restrictive filling.

Late diastolic antegrade flow in the PA is also a sign of restrictive filling; the high pressure produced in late diastole causes the pulmonary valve to open before systole and forward flow to occur. Measurement of RAP or right ventricular end-diastolic pressure (RVEDP) can be measured directly with right heart catheterization. Numerous studies have shown that the relationship between the right ventricular pressure and volume is not linear though. Further studies are needed to assess the specificity, sensitivity, and prognostic implications of diastolic dysfunction.

Physiology of chronic right heart strain: cor pulmonale

Cor pulmonale was originally a clinical diagnosis in an appropriate clinical context. With the advent of right heart catheterization, cor pulmonale was described as a central venous pressure higher than the PA occlusion pressure. In the modern era, cor pulmonale is now a clinical and echocardiographic diagnosis defined as the presence of right ventricular dilatation with paradoxical movement of the inter-ventricular septum in end-systole.

The key pathophysiological process of cor pulmonale is the laying down of extra parallel fibres and subsequent hypertrophy. The normal wall thickness of the RV is <5 mm. Chronic cor pulmonale is therefore associated with a thickened right ventricle (10–12 mm). This occurs

only very mildly in patients with acute cor pulmonale where, for example, slight thickening of the RV (5–6 mm) is seen within 3 days of starting mechanical ventilation.

It is the gradual right ventricular thickening and increase in right heart systolic and diastolic pressures which lead to two further key features of chronic cor pulmonale:

- Firstly, the RV is able to generate high-pressure TR jets of >60 mmHg which is not seen in acute cor pulmonale without prior conditioning of the RV. This can occur regardless of the size of the TR jet which is unrelated to its pressure in this setting. This is shown in Figure 4.15.

- Secondly, right ventricular hypertrophy maintains right ventricular structure until later on in cor pulmonale when the thickened ventricle begins to fail and dilate. Therefore, significant right ventricular dilatation should be considered to be a sign of acute cor pulmonale or late chronic cor pulmonale.

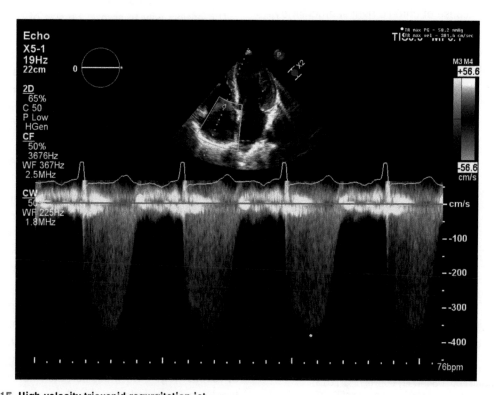

Figure 4.15 High-velocity tricuspid regurgitation jet.
© Oxford University Hospitals NHS Foundation Trust 2016, with permission.

Practice point

Looking at the dimensions of the RV is crucial to the differential diagnosis of acute and chronic right ventricular overload.

Thickening of the right ventricular free wall indicates adaptation to chronic increased afterload and is a key marker of chronic cor pulmonale.

High-pressure TR jets can only be generated by a conditioned RV.

In the chronic setting, right ventricular failure is an independent prognosticator in a number of conditions, including:

- Valvular heart disease
- Ischaemic and non-ischaemic cardiomyopathy
- PE
- Pulmonary arterial hypertension.

The causes of PHT are shown in Table 4.2 and reflect the most recent classification.

A common cause of chronic right ventricular dysfunction is left ventricular impairment or significant left heart valve disease leading to increased left atrial pressure. PHT is an important cause of right ventricular dysfunction. In 2003, a revised definition of the disease was introduced, classifying the

separate causes of the condition. Another important group that is becoming more common is right ventricular dysfunction due to congenital heart disease, for example tetralogy of Fallot, transposition of the great arteries, Ebstein's anomaly, and Eisenmenger syndrome.

The three key components of assessing the structure of the RV are:

- The size of the RV
- The thickness of the right ventricular free wall
- The relationship between the size of the RV and the LV, known as the eccentricity index (EI).

Right ventricular size

The RV increases in size in response to volume overload, pressure overload, and systolic failure. It is often the first sign of right ventricular dysfunction and is a prognostic indicator in patients with chronic pulmonary disease and acute PE. To produce an accurate measurement of the right ventricular size, its complex shape has to be considered.

The easiest way to assess the size of the RV is to qualitatively compare its size to the LV in the apical four-chamber view. It should be two-thirds the size of the LV. As it enlarges, it may also form the apex of the heart, displacing the LV from this position. In practice, this usually implies that the RV is at least moderately dilated, although this is not validated. These features are demonstrated in Figure 4.16.

The best correlation between single-plane, 2D right ventricular measurements and right ventricular volume measured using MRI is seen in the apical four-chamber view. There is a degree of overlap between normal and volume-overloaded conditions in mild to moderate enlargement, but in critical care we are looking for significant volume change in the right heart and referencing this against function.

The RV is optimally measured in the apical four-chamber view, with the focus adjusted onto the RV. Basal, mid-cavity, and longitudinal right ventricular measurements are obtained, termed as RVD1/2/3, respectively. Care must be taken not to overestimate or underestimate the right ventricular size through off-axis imaging. The plane of view should

Table 4.2 Causes of pulmonary hypertension

Groups	
1	Pulmonary arterial hypertension
2	Pulmonary venous hypertension
3	PHT due to hypoxia
4	Chronic thromboembolic PHT
5	Miscellaneous PHT

Adapted from *Journal of the American College of Cardiology*, 62, 25, Simonneau G., Gatzoulis, MA, Adatia I. et al., 'Updated clinical classification of pulmonary hypertension', pp. D34–D41, Copyright © 2013, with permission from American College of Cardiology Foundation.

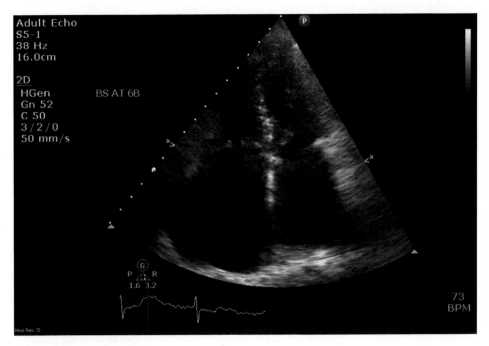

Figure 4.16 Right ventricular dilatation.
© Oxford University Hospitals NHS Foundation Trust 2016, with permission.

be through the apex and the centre of the left ventricular cavity. The LVOT must be closed, and the probe must be rotated to find the biggest plane view of the RV.

1. The basal diameter is defined as the largest short axis diameter in the basal one-third of the RV. In the normal RV, the biggest transverse diameter is in the basal third.

2. The mid-cavity diameter is measured in the middle third at the level of the left ventricular papillary muscles.

3. The longitudinal distance is measured from the apex of the RV to the plane of the tricuspid annulus.

Normal values are shown in Table 4.3.

Correlation with qualitative impression is very important when measuring the right ventricular dimensions. If the linear measurements are within the normal range, it remains valid to report the RV as dilated if it is larger than expected in relation to the LV.

Table 4.3 Reference limits for variables measured to assess right heart structure and function

Variable	Unit	Abnormal
Right ventricular basal diameter	cm	>4.2
Right ventricular mid diameter	cm	>3.5
Right ventricular longitudinal dimension	cm	>8.6
Right ventricular wall thickness	cm	>0.5
Right atrial end-systolic area	cm²	>18
TAPSE	cm	<1.6
Pulsed Doppler peak velocity at the annulus	cm/s	<10
Pulsed Doppler MPI	–	>0.40
Tissue Doppler MPI	–	>0.55
FAC	%	<0.35
Pulmonary acceleration time (PAT)	ms	<105

Right ventricular wall thickness

The RV is thin-walled in health but thickens in the presence of a chronic increase in afterload, hypertrophic cardiomyopathies, and infiltrative diseases. It is the single most important indicator of chronic cor pulmonale and therefore vitally important when trying to distinguish acute from chronic right ventricular stress.

Measurement of wall thickness can be performed by using the M-mode or 2D echocardiography in either the subcostal, parasternal, or apical windows. Wall thickness is usually measured in the subcostal view in end-diastole at the level of the tip of the anterior tricuspid valve leaflet. Care must be taken not to include trabeculations or papillary muscles in the measurement. The subcostal view has the least amount of variation and most closely correlates with the peak right ventricular systolic pressure. Right ventricular hypertrophy is present when the wall thickness is above 0.5 cm; there is no cut-off for an abnormally thin wall. Correct measurement of the right ventricular wall thickness is shown in Figure 4.17.

Eccentricity index

The RV shares the non-distensible pericardial compartment with the LV. As the RV dilates, the two chambers compete for space.

Normally, in an apical four-chamber view, the RV is around two-thirds the size of the LV.

As the RV dilates, the RV/LV ratio changes to:

- 0.8–1.0 in mild dilatation
- 1.1–1.4 in moderate dilatation
- >1.5 in severe right ventricular dilatation.

Dilatation of the RV can also be clearly seen in the parasternal short axis view. In this view, the LV has a circular cross-section. If there is right ventricular volume or pressure overload, then the septum becomes flattened and the LV becomes D-shaped.

- Predominantly volume overload is seen as left ventricular septal flattening in end-diastole, as the right ventricular pressure is increased relative to the LV
- Predominantly pressure overload is seen as left ventricular septal flattening in end-systole; as the

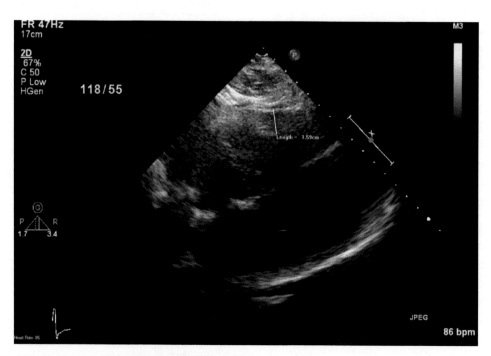

Figure 4.17 Measurement of right ventricular wall thickness.
© Oxford University Hospitals NHS Foundation Trust 2016, with permission.

Eccentricity index (EI)

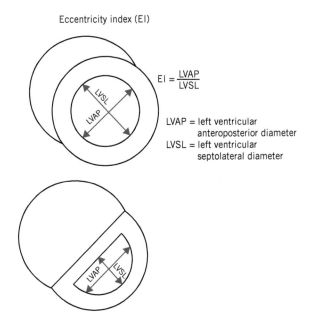

$$EI = \frac{LVAP}{LVSL}$$

LVAP = left ventricular
            anteroposterior diameter
LVSL = left ventricular
            septolateral diameter

Figure 4.18 Eccentricity index.

right ventricular pressure is increased, the right ventricular ejection time is prolonged.

The degree of flattening can be quantified using the EI (Figure 4.18). This is a measure of the parallel to perpendicular to left ventricular septum diameters, measured as shown in Figure 4.18 in the relevant cardiac phase. Normal range is 1.0, increasing to:

- 1.1–1.4 in mild
- 1.5–1.8 in moderate and
- >1.8 in severe septal bowing.

CASE STUDY

Acute cor pulmonale due to mechanical ventilation and subsequent management

A 60-year-old male was admitted to hospital with pneumonia. He was profoundly hypoxic and shocked; he was fluid-resuscitated in the emergency department, and his blood pressure improved. He was taken to the ICU and was intubated and started on mechanical ventilation. On his initial chest X-ray, he had bilateral changes consistent with acute respiratory distress syndrome. His ventilation was set up to achieve tidal volumes of 6 mL/kg with a high PEEP.

Over the course of the next days, he became hypotensive. He was further fluid-resuscitated and started on noradrenaline. His oxygenation improved over this time period, and the inspired oxygen concentration (FiO_2) was reduced. However, his noradrenaline requirement continued to increase.

An echocardiogram was performed which showed that he had a dilated RV with poor systolic function (TAPSE 11 mm). No TR jet could be found. In the parasternal short axis view, there was evidence of septal flattening both in systole and diastole. He was diagnosed with acute cor pulmonale.

The plateau pressure was measured which was 30 cmH$_2$O with a PEEP of 15. The FiO$_2$ was 0.50. It was decided to reduce the PEEP to 10, and this reduced the plateau pressure to 24 cmH$_2$O. The partial pressure of carbon dioxide (PaCO$_2$) was measured at 8.5 kPa. The respiratory rate was increased from 12 to 16 to reduce this.

A repeat echo was performed 12 hours later, showing a qualitative reduction in the degree of septal flattening and an improvement in the TAPSE.

CASE STUDY

Right heart anatomy aiding treatment limitation decisions

A 66-year-old female with chronic obstructive pulmonary disease was admitted to the A&E department with an acute exacerbation and a productive cough. Previously, she had been admitted the year before with a similar episode and had been successfully treated with NIV. Social history revealed that she had been living alone in a bungalow but, with help from her family, was still smoking and therefore had been turned down for long-term oxygen therapy.

A chest radiograph showed hyperexpanded lungs with no focal consolidation. The patient was initially treated with steroids, antibiotics, and nebulizers, and established on NIV. Following 48 hours of therapy, she developed worsening shortness of breath and low blood pressure. Her family were called in to discuss limitations of care since the patient was too drowsy to engage in this discussion.

An echocardiogram was performed to inform decision-making and demonstrated severe dilatation of the RV. The RV was also hypertrophied with a wall thickness of 9 mm,

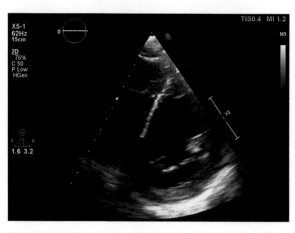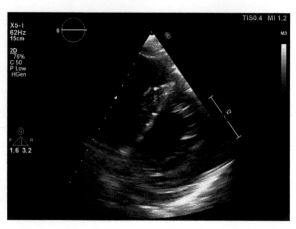

Figure 4.19 [Video 4.1] Septal collapse in diastole (left image) and systole (right image). The echo loop shows flattening of the septum thoughout the whole of the cardiac cycle.

This video is available t-o watch in the online video appendix.

© Oxford University Hospitals NHS Foundation Trust 2016, with permission.

and there was mild TR with a peak gradient of 70 mmHg. The PAT was measured at <80 ms. The TAPSE was reduced at 14 mm. There was evidence of septal collapse in both diastole and systole, as shown in Figure 4.19 .

The diagnosis of chronic cor pulmonale was discussed with the patient's family who agreed that intubation and ventilation and the use of vasopressors to support her blood pressure would not be appropriate or in her best interests. She was managed actively with NIV as the ceiling of care. After 12 hours on NIV, she became less drowsy, and 2 days later she was weaned off the NIV and was discharged to the ward.

Pulmonary embolism

The overall incidence of venous thromboembolism (VTE) is 1–3 cases per 1000 per year. This rate increases as age does, so the risk of VTE when aged >50 is 1 in 100.

Clinically acute PE is defined as massive, sub-massive, or non-massive. Haemodynamic stability and right ventricular function are crucially important in determining morbidity and mortality.

- Massive PE is defined as systemic hypotension with a systolic pressure <90 mmHg, shock, or cardiac arrest. A massive PE has an estimated 60% mortality within the first hour after onset.

- Sub-massive PE is defined by normotension with imaging or enzyme evidence of right ventricular dysfunction. Sub-massive PE has an associated 30-day mortality of 15–20% but also has been associated with development of cor pulmonale secondary to chronic thromboembolic PHT.

- Non-massive PE is defined by normotension without evidence of right ventricular dysfunction.

Acute PE leads to an acute rise in PVR. There is a possibility that a pro-inflammatory state develops within the RV too, compromising right ventricular function. Although TTE may not offer true anatomic approximations of the RV, it does give information on those patients at risk of deterioration. Outcome is dependent on clot burden, which can be quantified using CT pulmonary angiography (CTPA); aside from this, cardiac reserve is also important. Some patients with a massive PE but good cardiac reserve will behave the same as those with a smaller clot burden but with less cardiac reserve.

Right ventricular dilatation, assessed by echocardiography, is present in ≥25% of patients with PE. A number of echocardiographic parameters correlate with the clot burden and right ventricular dysfunction. An RV–LV diameter ratio >0.9, a TR max pressure gradient, PAT, and TAPSE all indicate right ventricular dysfunction if >25% of the pulmonary vascular tree is obstructed. The 60–60 sign is an echocardiographic finding showing a disturbed ejection pattern. This is the presence of a PAT of <60 ms, but in conjunction with a TR pressure gradient of <60 mmHg. The McConnell's sign is the presence of a regional right ventricular dysfunction with apical sparing. Originally thought to be pathognomonic of PE, it has subsequently been shown that the McConnell's sign is less reliable, as this pattern has been demonstrated in patients with acute right ventricular infarction. Echocardiography may also show right-to-left shunting through a patent foramen ovale and the presence of right heart thrombi, which are both associated with increased mortality.

In those with a massive PE, thrombolytic therapy has been shown to resolve the obstructing thrombus and reduce the PVR, increasing the right ventricular cardiac output. TTE can aid in diagnosis when a CT scan is not available but also can help diagnose other potential causes of shock, for example tamponade, acute valvular dysfunction, or severe left ventricular dysfunction. In some cases, TTE may identify the presence of right ventricular hypertrophy or a TR jet velocity of such high velocity it would be incompatible with acute right ventricular pressure overload. For these cases, chronic PHT and chronic thromboembolic PHT should be entertained as differential diagnoses. The benefit of thrombolysis in those patients with sub-massive PE is less clear; the presence of a raised mortality rate is not consistent across all studies. Meta-analyses show that echocardiographic right ventricular dysfunction is associated with an increased short-term mortality in haemodynamically stable patients.

Those in this intermediate-risk group warrant further assessment. Individuals who have echocardiographic evidence of right ventricular dysfunction and elevated cardiac biomarkers should be classified into an intermediate- to high-risk group and would benefit from close monitoring to permit early detection of haemodynamic demise necessitating rescue reperfusion therapy (Figure 4.20).

Propofol-related infusion syndrome

Propofol-related infusion syndrome (PRIS) is a rare drug-related complication and carries a high mortality.

It was first reported in paediatric populations in the 1990s. It has subsequently been reported in adult populations, particularly in critically ill patients, since then. Due to the rarity of the condition, the pathophysiology is still unclear and understanding of the disease is limited to case reports and small case series.

The clinical features include bradycardia, cardiovascular collapse with dysrhythmias, high anion gap metabolic acidosis, rhabdomyolysis, hepatomegaly, and lipaemia. It is thought that propofol uncouples oxidative phosphorylation and energy production in mitochondria. In stress conditions, there is a shift to using free fatty acids as a major source of energy for biological tissues maintained by the stress hormones cortisol and adrenaline. Propofol inhibits the mitochondrial enzyme carnitine palmitoyl transferase 1 which leads to an accumulation of acylcarnitine and fatty acids in various organs. These have been shown to promote cardiac arrhythmogenicity. Propofol also antagonizes beta adrenoceptor binding and inhibits cardiac L-type calcium currents, leading to diminished cardiac contractility and increased inflammation in the cardiac muscle. Patients with PRIS therefore have decreased energy availability at a time of increased metabolic demand. This may explain the observed myocytolysis of both skeletal and cardiac muscles in patients with PRIS.

A typical presentation is the formation of a Brugada-like ECG pattern (coved-type ST elevation in leads V1–V3), ventricular tachyarrhythmias, dilatation of the right heart, and severe right heart failure and asystole. The only case report to serially track the progression of the disease showed an acute right heart failure with dilatation, with preserved left-sided systolic function. These right-sided changes resolved rapidly after cessation of propofol.

Treatment involves immediate cessation of propofol with advanced cardiovascular support. The use of phosphodiesterase inhibitors, glucagon, and calcium may be beneficial in augmenting cardiovascular performance, given the effect of propofol on calcium channels and catecholamine-binding sites. In extreme cases, extracorporeal mechanical support should be considered.

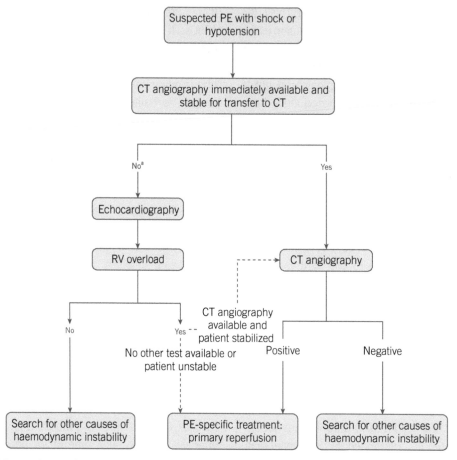

Figure 4.20 Diagnostic algorithm for patients with suspected high-risk PE. [a]Includes cases in which the patient's condition is so critical that it only allows bedside diagnostic tests.

Reproduced from SV Konstantinides et al., '2014 ESC Guidelines on the Diagnosis and Management of Acute Pulmonary Embolism', *European Heart Journal*, 2014, 35, 43, pp. 3033–3080, by permission of European Society of Cardiology

CASE STUDY

Pulmonary embolism and risk stratification

A 25-year-old lady was admitted to hospital with a 4-day history of intermittent chest pain. That morning, she came to the emergency department with a recurrence of the pain again, but this time it was associated with a feeling of light-headedness. She underwent a CTPA and high-volume bilateral PEs were diagnosed.

On returning from the CT scanner, her systolic blood pressure dropped to 80 mmHg and responded to 500 mL of intravenous fluid. An echocardiogram was performed. The RV was moderately dilated with a normal TAPSE. No TR jet could be found, but the PAT was measured at 80 ms. In the

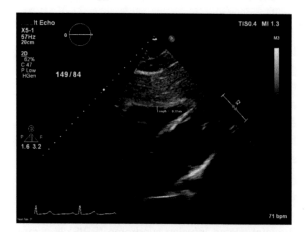

Figure 4.21 Right ventricular free wall <5 mm thick.
© Oxford University Hospitals NHS Foundation Trust 2016, with permission.

short axis view, there was flattening of the septum in systole. The thickness of the right ventricular wall was normal at <5 mm (Figure 4.21).

The echocardiogram demonstrated no signs of chronic PHT; however, there was an element of acute right heart dysfunction, although not yet impacting longitudinal function. The low PAT was consistent with raised PVR and a useful marker of severity of illness in the absence of a TR jet.

The patient was therapeutically anticoagulated and admitted to a high-dependency bed for invasive blood pressure monitoring.

Multiple choice questions

1. The following are consistent with good right ventricular systolic function:
   A TAPSE of 18 mm
   B dP/dT of 300 mmHg
   C Myocardial performance index using TDi of 0.60
   D Right ventricular fractional area change of 30%
   E Right ventricular ejection fraction of 50%

2. Regarding right ventricular anatomy:
   A The right ventricle is made up of the inflow, conus, and infundibulum
   B The end-diastolic volume of the right ventricle is usually greater than that of the left ventricle
   C The right ventricle is only supplied by the right coronary artery
   D The most superficial muscle fibres of the right ventricle are arranged longitudinally
   E The right ventricle has a triangular cross-section at the apex

3. Which of the following measurements are consistent with a dilated right ventricle?
   A The right ventricle forms the apex of the heart
   B There is septal flattening in diastole
   C The longitudinal dimension is 80 mm
   D The mid-level dimension is 42 mm
   E The right ventricle measures within the normal range but is bigger than the left ventricle

4. Right ventricular physiology:
   A The right ventricle is perfused throughout all of the cardiac cycle
   B A pulmonary artery systolic pressure of 25 mmHg is consistent with pulmonary hypertension
   C The right ventricle has a lower ejection fraction than the left ventricle
   D Right ventricular ejection is almost totally provided by contraction of the free wall
   E The pulmonary arteries are more compliant than the aorta

5. Regarding pulmonary embolism:
   A Young people are more at risk than the elderly
   B A tricuspid valve pressure gradient of 80 mmHg is explained by an acute pulmonary embolism
   C A pulmonary acceleration time of 60 ms is consistent with raised pulmonary vascular resistance
   D It is possible to rule out a pulmonary embolism in a shocked patient using echocardiography
   E The McConnell's sign is pathognomonic for pulmonary embolism

For answers to multiple choice questions, please see 'Appendix 1: Answers to multiple choice questions', p. 171.

Further reading

Karas MG, Kizer JR. Echocardiographic assessment of the right ventricle and associated hemodynamics. *Prog Cardiovasc Dis* 2012; **55**: 144–60.

Konstantinides SV, Torbicki A, Agnelli G, *et al.*; Task Force for the Diagnosis and Management of Acute Pulmonary Embolism of the European Society of Cardiology (ESC). 2014 ESC guidelines on the diagnosis and management of acute pulmonary embolism. *Eur Heart J* 2014; **35**: 3033–80.

Mitoff PR, Beauchesne L, Dick AJ, *et al.* Imaging the failing right ventricle. *Curr Opin Cardiol* 2012; **27**: 148–53.

Rudski LG, Lai WW, Afilalo J, *et al.* Guidelines for the echocardiographic assessment of the right heart in adults: a report from the American Society of Echocardiography endorsed by the European Association of Echocardiography, a registered branch of the European Society of Cardiology, and the Canadian Society of Echocardiography. *J Am Soc Echocardiogr* 2010; **23**: 685–713.

Tan TC, Hung J. Role of echocardiography in the assessment of right heart disease: update 2013. *Curr Cardiovasc Imaging Rep* 2013; **6**: 486–97.

5

Valve disease in critical illness

Aortic stenosis

Definition, aetiology, and prevalence

Aortic stenosis (AS) is the most common valvular heart disease in Europe and North America and is characterized by obstruction of blood flow from the LV. The obstruction is typically due to valvular degeneration with chronic calcification of a normal tri-leaflet valve but, in rare cases, can be due to supra- or subvalvular pathology. The prevalence of AS is 0.2% amongst adults aged 50–59 years, rising to 2.8% in people aged over 70 years.

A bicuspid aortic valve, present in 1–2% of the population, accounts for 60% of aortic valve replacements in patient <70 years of age. Rheumatic AS is rare in the developed world and is usually accompanied by mitral valve disease. Figure 5.1 shows the classic orientations of a bicuspid aortic valve with fusion of a median raphe between two leaflets.

Pathophysiology

Degenerative AS has a long latent period and starts with mild leaflet thickening without a haemodynamic effect (aortic sclerosis) to valve obstruction. Progressive fibrosis, and then calcification, occurs initially at the base of the cusps, then across the whole leaflet. Stenosis develops slowly, with an average peak transvalvular velocity increase of 0.1–0.3 m/s per year and a reduction in valve area by 0.1 cm² per year.

Increases in left ventricular pressure required to overcome the valvular stenosis cause increased wall thickness or hypertrophy whereby the muscle fibre diameter and the total collagen volume fraction increase, and interstitial fibrosis occurs. These structural and pressure changes of the LV reduce its compliance, causing diastolic dysfunction and then secondary PHT. The high end-diastolic pressures impair subendocardial blood flow, which, along with the increased oxygen demand of the hypertrophied LV, can cause ischaemia, even in the absence of coronary artery disease, although 30–50% of patients with degenerative AS do have concomitant coronary atherosclerosis. Eventually, a point is reached where no further compensatory hypertrophy of the LV can occur, and the LV fails with a dilated cavity and a reduction in the EF.

The mortality from AS in patients with symptomatic disease is 50% at 2 years.

Echocardiographic assessment of aortic stenosis

TTE is the key diagnostic tool; however, grading AS can be complex. The role of echocardiography is to confirm the presence of AS and to assess for any calcification, the number of leaflets, left ventricular function and wall thickness, and any associated valvular disease. Doppler echocardiography is the preferred technique for evaluating the severity of AS, as transvalvular pressure gradients are flow-dependent. Planimetry is not routinely performed to measure the aortic valve area, as the calcified and irregular orifice is hard to measure accurately and is often overestimated.

PLAX

In the PLAX view, the aortic valve is bisected with an anterior right coronary cusp and the non-coronary cusp posteriorly. Figure 5.2 shows normal opening and reduced opening in a normal and stenotic valve,

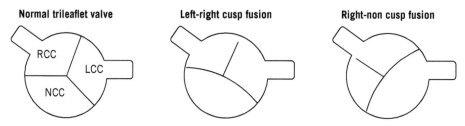

Figure 5.1 **Normal trileaflet aortic valve and orientation of leaflet fusion in bicuspid valves.**

respectively. M-mode demonstrations are also shown. Look for a central closure line in the M-mode view. An eccentric closure line and doming of the aortic valve cusps as the valve opens suggest a bicuspid aortic valve.

Optimize the LV and freeze the image. Scroll back to the end of diastole and measure the interventricular septum (IVSd), left ventricular internal diameter (LVIDd), and posterior wall (PWd). Ensure the measurement is orthogonal to the long axis of the LV (Figure 5.3). Normal and abnormal values are shown in Table 5.1.

Zoom over the aortic valve, and carefully measure the LVOT diameter in mid systole, inner edge to inner edge, just below the aortic valve orifice—it is usually 1.8–2.2 cm. The area can be calculated by πr^2. The correct position for measurement is shown in Figure 5.4.

Also place the colour box over the aortic valve, and assess for any associated aortic regurgitation (AR) or subvalvular or valvular turbulent flow.

PSAX

In the PSAX, an assessment should be made of the number of cusps. In addition, fusion and calcification of the cusps can be described. Place the colour box over the aortic valve, and assess for any associated regurgitation which will be seen as a colour jet coming towards you. Figure 5.5 ◖◗ shows normal tricuspid anatomy.

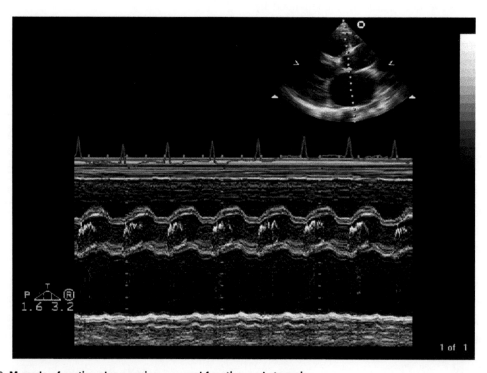

Figure 5.2 **M-mode of aortic valve opening—normal function and stenosis.**

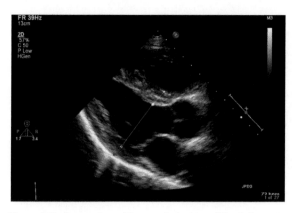

Figure 5.3 A parasternal long axis image of the left ventricle frozen at end-diastole and the wall thickness and cavity size measured.

© Oxford University Hospitals NHS Foundation Trust 2016, with permission.

Peak velocity and mean pressure gradient

The severity of AS can be gauged from the peak velocity, the mean pressure gradient, and the aortic valve area, which is derived from the continuity equation. From the apical five-chamber position, place the continuous-wave (CW) Doppler through the aortic valve into the aorta. Observe the spectral trace which measures the velocity of the forward flow of blood through the aorta. In severe AS, the peak of the spectral trace occurs in mid systole. Freeze the image, and measure the spectral trace with the greatest (peak) velocity (AV_{max}).

Next, trace the envelope of the CW spectral trace. The echo machine software package will generate the mean pressure gradient and the velocity time integral (VTI). The VTI is the area underneath the curve and represents the total flow. Peak velocity and VTI measurements are shown in Figure 5.6.

These measurements are derived from flow across the aortic valve. Therefore, where there is increased flow, such as AR or pregnancy, the degree of AS can be overestimated; conversely, decreased flow is associated with underestimation of the severity of AS.

Continuity equation

The continuity equation is based upon the principle that, for a non-compressible fluid, the product of the cross-sectional area and flow velocity must be constant and is therefore a relatively **flow-independent** measure of AS.

Place the pulsed-wave (PW) Doppler in the LVOT, and review the spectral trace. Freeze the image with the most defined and highest velocity peak. Trace the envelope to obtain the peak velocity ($LVOT_{max}$) and the VTI. Take care not to place the sample volume too close to the aortic valve, as this will record flow in the convergence zone and overestimate the valve area.

$$AV_{area} \times AV_{VTI} = LVOT_{area} \times LVOT_{VTI}$$

Rearranged:

$$AV_{area} = LVOT_{area} \times LVOT_{VTI} / AV_{VTI}$$

Dimensionless index

Another simple Doppler assessment is to derive the ratio of LVOT flow to aortic flow by dividing the $LVOT_{VTI}$ by the AV_{VTI} (Table 5.2). This produces an index of severity that does not rely on assessment of the LVOT cross-sectional area but is a flow-dependent parameter.

Table 5.1 Normal and abnormal values for left ventricular wall thickness and chamber size

	Normal	Mild	Moderate	Severe
Left ventricular wall thickness IVSd/PWd (cm)	0.6–1.2	1.3–1.5	1.6–1.9	≥2.0
LVIDd, women (cm)	3.9–5.3	5.4–5.7	5.8–6.1	≥6.2
LVIDd, men (cm)	4.2–5.9	6.0–6.3	6.4–6.8	≥6.9

Zoomed image frozen in mid systole

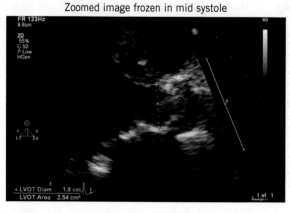

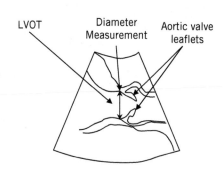

Figure 5.4 Measuring the left ventricular outflow tract diameter in mid systole.

5.4a = © Oxford University Hospitals NHS Foundation Trust 2016, with permission.

Practice point

Take care to measure the LVOT diameter and $LVOT_{VTI}$ as accurately as possible, as small errors are magnified by the equation and it is easy to overestimate the severity of the stenosis. If possible, also measure the peak velocity through the aortic valve from different windows to ensure the true peak velocity has not been underestimated.

Left ventricular function and aortic stenosis

Ultimately, left ventricular function worsens with AS. With left ventricular dysfunction, lower flows are generated across the aortic valve. Any echocardiographic measurement that is dependent on flow, such as peak and mean Doppler gradients, will therefore underestimate the severity of AS in the presence of left ventricular dysfunction.

Effect of stroke volume on measured parameters of aortic stenosis

In patients with poor left ventricular function and visibly abnormal aortic valves, it can be challenging to accurately determine the severity of the stenosis. The continuity equation may give a valve area in the severely stenosed range, but the measured gradients may only be in the moderate, or even the

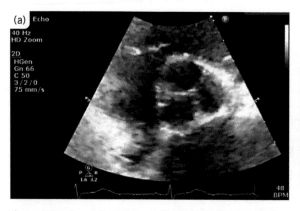

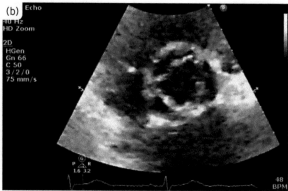

Figure 5.5 (a) and (b) [Video 5.1] Normal trileaflet aortic valve from the parasternal short axis position.

🔘 *This video is available to watch in the online video appendix.*

5.5a = © Oxford University Hospitals NHS Foundation Trust 2016, with permission.

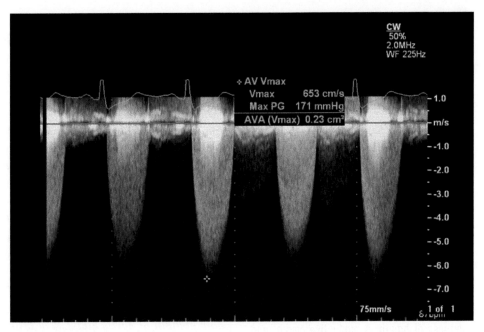

Figure 5.6 Continuous-wave Doppler flow through the outflow tract in a patient with critical aortic stenosis—peak pressure gradient of 171 mmHg.

© Oxford University Hospitals NHS Foundation Trust 2016, with permission.

mild, range. In some cases, this is because the AS is truly severe and the LV has failed as a result—the continuity equation is correct and the low gradients are a reflection of reduced SV. Conversely, in some patients, left ventricular function is poor for other reasons, and although the valve is abnormal, it is not severely stenosed; however, it appears to open poorly and the continuity equation gives a small orifice area, as the valve is not being opened fully by the reduced SV.

The best way to determine the relationship of flow and AS severity in these cases is to improve left ventricular function and increase SV by administering a positive inotropic agent, typically dobutamine. In true severe stenosis, the left ventricular function should improve and SV increases, but as the AS is fixed and severe, the valve gradients will climb, but the valve area derived by the continuity equation will remain the same or even fall. In non-severe cases, the valve area will increase as the SV climbs and the valve is opened to its full amount.

Table 5.2 Severity grading of aortic stenosis derived from Doppler measurements

	Normal	Mild	Moderate	Severe
Peak velocity (m/s)	–	<2.9	3–3.9	>4.0
Mean pressure drop (mmHg)	–	<25	25–40	>40
AV area (cm²)	>2	1.5–2.0	1.0–1.4	<1.0
Dimensionless index	–	0.5	0.25–0.5	<0.25

Adapted from Helmut Baumgartner et al., 'Echocardiographic assessment of valve stenosis: EAE/ASE recommendations for clinical practice', *European Heart Journal: Cardiovascular Imaging*, 10, pp. 1–25, Copyright The Author 2008.

Practice point

In critically ill patients, be vigilant when categorizing the severity of AS and ensure abnormalities in left ventricular function or SV are integrated into the assessment of valve function—a patient can have critical AS with a peak velocity of only 3 m/s if left ventricular function is very poor.

CASE STUDY

Aortic stenosis complicating the presentation of pneumonia

A 58-year-old man presented to the emergency department with acute shortness of breath, a productive cough, and fevers of 4 days' duration. He had a past medical history of hypertension, for which he took ramipril 2.5 mg once daily. He was a non-smoker and non-drinker and normally became short of breath on moderate exertion.

On assessment, he was hypotensive (blood pressure 84/50, mean arterial pressure (MAP) 61 mmHg), tachycardic at 104 bpm, and tachypnoeic at 32 breaths per minute, with oxygen saturations of 91% on 15 L oxygen via a non-rebreathe mask. His bloods revealed increased inflammatory markers C-reactive protein (CRP) 254 mg/L and white cell count (WCC) 17.5×10^9/L, normal haematology and liver function tests, and an acute kidney injury (AKI) with urea 13 mmol/L and creatinine 150 mmol/L. His ECG showed LVH with a strain pattern, and his chest radiograph showed right basal consolidation.

Due to his increased work of breathing and type 1 respiratory failure with a pO_2 of 7.4 kPa, he was intubated in the emergency department and transferred to the ICU. Low-dose noradrenaline was started initially at 0.05 micrograms/kg/min following 2 L of crystalloid resuscitation, and he remained sedated on propofol and fentanyl. Within 4 hours, noradrenaline was escalated to maintain an MAP of >65 mmHg, and at a noradrenaline dose of 0.5 micrograms/kg/min, he became haemodynamically unstable with a tachycardia of 130 bpm and ischaemic changes on his rhythm strip. Peripherally, he was cool and mottled.

TTE was used to assess his cardiac function in the context of progressive hypotension. The main findings were moderate LVH, a normal-sized but hyperdynamic LV, and a calcified aortic valve with an aortic valve area calculated by the continuity equation of 0.9 cm². The IVC showed >50% collapse on full ventilation.

In light of the echo findings, he was given boluses of 250 mL of crystalloid to a total of 2 L and a unit of blood to achieve a target of >10 g/L. His sedation was changed to morphine and midazolam, and the noradrenaline was weaned to 0.12 micrograms/kg/min. Within 2 hours, he became normotensive and the ischaemic ECG resolved. Following extubation, his valve area was re-assessed and he was referred to cardiology services for consideration of urgent aortic valve replacement.

Management of aortic stenosis in critical care

Practice point

- Aortic valve disease is a fixed valve lesion, and the aperture for ejection cannot be altered, except by surgery.
- Maintaining cardiac output relies on maintaining the 'status quo' in relation to both SVR and cardiac work.
- Artificially increasing cardiac work using inotropes will increase the gradient and thereby REDUCE cardiac output, negatively affecting limb and organ perfusion.
- The response to over-vasoconstriction will be tachycardia, the net result of which will be to reduce coronary filling time, generating ischaemia in a predisposed ventricle and reducing cardiac output by reducing left ventricular filling time.

Therefore:

- Avoid moderate to large doses of any inotrope or vasopressor
- Low-dose vasopressors may be useful to maintain a constant SVR against sedative drugs
- Ensure adequate oxygenation, haemoglobin, and fluid volumes

- Where over-volume resuscitation has occurred into a ventricle with high filling pressures, **careful** off-loading may improve cardiac output
- Normalize the temperature
- Take over high work of breathing where this is present
- Avoid sedative drugs with a potent cardiovascular impact
- Avoid any drug causing a tachycardia
- Have a low threshold for the aggressive maintenance of sinus rhythm where arrhythmias occur
- In rare cases, aortic valve replacement or valvuloplasty may be essential before the patient can be weaned from ventilation.

Mitral stenosis

Definition, aetiology, and prevalence

Mitral stenosis (MS) occurs when the mitral valve (MV) leaflets become immobile and thickened, obstructing blood flow from the LA to the LV. It remains common in the developing world because of the relatively high incidence of rheumatic fever (RF). MS is now an uncommon valve lesion in non-immigrant UK residents due to the eradication of RF. In the elderly, functional stenosis due to progressive annular calcification of the MV annulus does occur. The prevalence of MS detected by echocardiography in developed countries is 0.02–0.2%.

Other rare causes include congenital abnormalities, inflammatory diseases such as rheumatoid arthritis, post-mitral valve surgery, or in the setting of abnormal serotonin metabolism.

Pathophysiology

The normal MV area is 4–6 cm² and has no measurable gradient when open. The classical findings of rheumatic MV disease are thickening and fusion of the MV commissural edges and chordae, resulting in a 'hockey-stick' shape to the open anterior MV leaflet. Normal and rheumatic valves seen in the PLAX view are seen in Figure 5.7 ◖.

In rheumatic heart disease, the MV is involved in 80% of cases. Resistance to blood flow occurs due to the narrowing, which may be compounded by chordal fusion and shortening as the disease progresses.

The haemodynamic consequence of this is the creation of a pressure gradient between the LA and LV in diastole. The LA becomes grossly enlarged in long-standing disease. PHT is a common complication of MS due to the backward transmission of elevated left atrial pressures. The consequences of PHT include

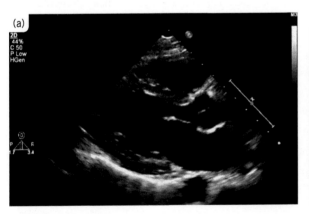
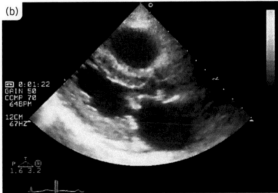

Figures 5.7 (a) [Video 5.2] and 5.7 (b) [Video 5.3] Parasternal long axis view of a normal and rheumatic mitral valve.

◖ These videos are available to watch in the online video appendix.

5.7a = © Oxford University Hospitals NHS Foundation Trust 2016, with permission.

right ventricular hypertrophy and enlargement, TR, increased right atrial pressure, and eventually right heart failure. A third of patients have associated systolic dysfunction. Diastolic dysfunction is also associated with MS due to impaired chamber compliance.

Echocardiographic assessment

MV structure and morphology should be carefully assessed to determine the cause, alongside haemodynamic consequences of valve narrowing to determine the severity. Severity of MS should be defined by several corroborative measurements. Current guidelines recommend MV planimetry at the narrowest point of the valve, and pressure half-time ($P_{1/2}$) or pressure gradient across the MV.

Appearance

The appearance of the MV can be observed best in the PLAX and PSAX views, with emphasis on:

- Leaflet mobility and shape in diastole
- Leaflet thickening and calcification; >5 mm is abnormal
- Annular calcification, suggesting non-rheumatic MS
- Subvalvular involvement of the chordae and attachments
- Look for associated features of MS, including right heart disease.

Mitral valve area

In the PSAX view, angle the image to show the tips of the leaflets at maximal excursion. Record a loop, and scroll to locate the point of maximal opening in diastole. The entire MV orifice should be visualized in a single image or the measurement will be inaccurate. The inner edge of the MV orifice can then be traced and the valve area measured, as shown in Figure 5.8.

Limitations

This measurement is relatively independent of haemodynamic factors but can underestimate the severity of disease, especially in moderate to severe MS, because it relies on perfect geometric alignment. Modern echocardiography platforms capable of 3D imaging can overcome this, as perfect alignment with the tips of the MV can be ensured.

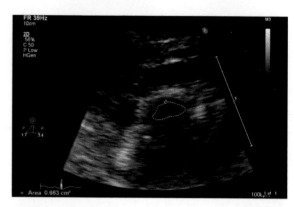

Figure 5.8 Zoomed parasternal short axis view of the tips of the mitral valve.
© Oxford University Hospitals NHS Foundation Trust 2016, with permission.

Pressure half-time (ms)

This is complimentary to 2D planimetry and measures the time taken for the transmitral pressure to halve from its peak value. In the apical four-chamber view (A4C), align continuous-wave Doppler with the colour inflow jet, and minimize any incident angle between the Doppler calliper and jet. Record a spectral trace, as shown in Figure 5.9. The E wave represents passive left ventricular filling, and the A wave, absent in AF, represents atrial systole. Use the slope of the E wave to calculate the $P_{1/2}$.

If the slope has two gradients, trace the flatter of the two. Measure from point to point on the flat part of the slope. In patients with AF, take several measurements in long diastoles and average the measurements.

The relationship between the mitral valve area (MVA) and $P_{1/2}$ is as follows:

$$MVA\ (cm^2) = 220 / P_{1/2}\ (ms)$$

Mean gradient (mmHg)

Using the same image, also trace round the Doppler diastolic mitral flow profile, as shown in Figure 5.9. The mean and maximum gradients will be calculated by the machine, based on the formula:

$$Pressure\ gradient = 4 \times velocity^2$$

See Table 5.3 for the severity grading of MS using these echo parameters.

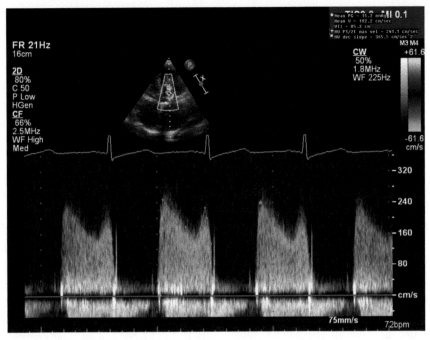

Figure 5.9 Transmitral Doppler from the apical four-chamber position, with pressure half-time and mean gradient measured.

© Oxford University Hospitals NHS Foundation Trust 2016, with permission.

Limitations

- $P_{1/2}$ is affected by abnormal left atrial or left ventricular compliance.

- High resting left ventricular pressure, for example in LVH or coexistent significant AR, will shorten the $P_{1/2}$ and overestimate the valve area.

- An atrial septal defect (ASD) that off-loads blood from the LA into the right atrium during transmitral filling will also artificially shorten the $P_{1/2}$, increasing the calculated valve area.

Reasons for decompensation

Symptoms of breathlessness and fatigue generally start when the MVA is <1.5 cm². MS is a fixed cardiac output state; therefore, patients with moderate or worse MS have minimal reserve in situations where cardiac output is augmented by volume or where there is a change in cardiac rate and rhythm such as sepsis or pregnancy.

Other ways in which patients may present to critical care include:

- Haemoptysis due to PHT and vascular congestion or sudden haemorrhage due to rupture of the dilated and thin-walled bronchial veins

Table 5.3 Severity grading of mitral stenosis derived from echocardiographic measurements

	Normal	Mild	Moderate	Severe
MVA (cm²)	4.0–6.0	1.6–2.0	1.0–1.5	<1.0
MV $P_{1/2}$ (ms)	40–70	71–139	140–219	>220
Mean pressure gradient (mmHg)		<5	5–10	>10

Adapted from Helmut Baumgartner et al., 'Echocardiographic assessment of valve stenosis: EAE/ASE recommendations for clinical practice', *European Heart Journal: Cardiovascular Imaging*, 10, pp. 1–25, Copyright The Author 2008.

- Thromboembolism: most commonly cerebral due to AF, low or reduced cardiac output, and dilated LA and appendage
- Infective endocarditis (IE)
- Right-sided heart failure, which may also be precipitated by intubation and ventilation for other presentations

Importance of rate control and filling

Tachycardia is detrimental in MS, as the reduction in diastole leads to reduced left ventricular filling time and increased left atrial pressure, accentuating right heart strain and precipitating pulmonary oedema. The active phase of diastolic filling of the LV is critical to maintaining cardiac output. When AF occurs, this is lost, frequently causing abrupt deterioration and increasing symptoms.

When AF occurs acutely, it should be rate-controlled with beta blockers or calcium channel blockers; restoration of sinus rhythm is the ultimate aim, but this may be difficult in the face of severe left atrial enlargement.

MS with AF carries an annual risk of embolic stroke of 7–15% per annum. Formal anticoagulation with warfarin is indicated with a target international normalized ratio (INR) of 2.5–3.5. Patients in sinus rhythm with a history of VTE should also be anticoagulated.

Mechanical relief of the obstruction—with either balloon mitral valvotomy (BMV) or surgical MV replacement—is the only definitive therapy.

Practice point

Significant MS is extremely poorly tolerated in the setting of critical illness. Careful consideration must be given to early valvotomy as part of critical care therapy if the patient is in intractable pulmonary oedema.

CASE STUDY

Surgical intervention to the mitral valve during cardiovascular stress

A 27-year-old primigravida from Mozambique presented to the emergency department at 24 weeks' gestation with shortness of breath. She was in sinus rhythm with a heart rate of 110 bpm, blood pressure of 96/40, and MAP of 59 mmHg. On auscultation of her chest, she had a diastolic murmur graded 4/6 in the mitral area and bibasal fine inspiratory crepitations. Her bloods showed a normocytic anaemia with haemoglobin (Hb) of 10 g/dL. The remainder of her full blood count and renal function were normal. An ECG was recorded which showed p-mitrale and right ventricular hypertrophy. A chest X-ray showed evidence of pulmonary oedema.

TTE demonstrated MS (Figure 5.10 📹) with an MVA of 1.0 cm with a $P_{1/2}$ of 200 ms and a mean pressure gradient of 10 mmHg. She also had evidence of PHT.

Initial management consisted of transfer to a critical care area for labetolol infusion, careful offloading with 20 mg of intravenous furosemide, and treatment with therapeutic low-molecular-weight heparin to prevent stroke. However, despite bed rest, her symptoms became progressive, and at 28 weeks she underwent a BMV. This improved the MVA to 1.6 cm² and the mean gradient to 5 mmHg, and the remainder of the pregnancy proceeded uneventfully.

Mitral and aortic regurgitation in intensive care

Introduction

The effects of valvular regurgitation on the cardiovascular system depend on the speed of onset, the presence of comorbidities, and the interventions initiated, as shown in Table 5.4. Most regurgitant lesions are chronic and slowly progressive. Cardiac remodelling in chronic lesions is compensatory and aims to maintain normal cardiac output; volume loading leads to progressive hypertrophy and dilatation and increased SV to compensate for the regurgitation. With acute lesions, abrupt decompensation can occur. Clarification of the mechanism and rate of development of the lesion is essential to guide management and prognosis.

Aortic regurgitation

Anatomy

The aortic valve is a tri-leaflet outflow valve separating the LV from the aorta. The base of each leaflet insertion, despite the absence of an anatomically or

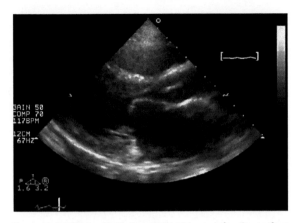

Figure 5.10 [Video 5.4] Parasternal long axis of a patient with MS presenting in pregnancy.

🎥 *This video is available to watch in the online video appendix.*
© Oxford University Hospitals NHS Foundation Trust 2016, with permission.

histologically distinct circular structure, is nominally referred to as the **annulus**. Each leaflet (or **cusp**) is of similar size and carries a small nodule on its tip (**nodule of Arantius**). Upstream of each cusp is the **sinus of Valsalva**—an outpouching of the aortic root from which the coronary arteries originate. Cusps and associated sinuses are named according to the artery that emerges from the sinus (right, left, and non).

Above the valve, the sinuses merge with the tubular ascending aorta at the **sinotubular junction**. Together, the cusps, sinuses, annulus, and junction make up the **aortic root**. Below the valve is the **left ventricular outflow tract** consisting of the membranous interventricular septum, the anterior mitral valve leaflet (aMVL), and the anterior left ventricular wall.

Aetiology

AR results from inadequate leaflet coaptation, due to pathology of the leaflets, the aortic root, or both. Causes of chronic AR include valvular degeneration and aortic root dilation (with or without a bicuspid valve), rheumatic heart disease, and connective tissue or rheumatologic disorders. Aortic root dilation is the most common cause and is typically idiopathic.

Acute AR is most often due to IE but may also occur with leaflet rupture following blunt trauma or aortic dissection of any aetiology. Causes may overlap—for instance, a bicuspid valve may induce chronic AR through both leaflet pathology and progressive root dilation, and acute AR via aortic dissection. Chronic regurgitation is usually well tolerated, whereas acute regurgitation often leads to rapid cardiovascular decompensation.

Acute severe AR is a surgical emergency, but accurate and timely diagnosis can be problematic. Examination findings to suggest acute AR (in contrast to chronic AR) may be subtle, and the clinical presentation may be non-specific. Consequently, acute AR may be mistaken for other acute conditions

Table 5.4 Factors influencing the haemodynamic effect of regurgitant lesions

Dominant lesion	Regurgitation vs stenosis
Speed of onset	Acute vs chronic
Underlying disease	Ischaemia, hypertension, or LVH
Arrhythmias	AF
Comorbidities	Pulmonary disease affecting right heart lesions
Presenting illness	Sepsis, hypervolaemia
Interventions	Anaesthesia, positive pressure ventilation, vasopressors, or inotropes

Adapted from Newton J, Sabharwal N, Myerson S et al., *Oxford Specialist Handbooks in Cardiology: Valvular Heart Disease*, 2011, p. 4, with permission from Oxford University Press

such as sepsis, pneumonia, or non-valvular heart failure.

Pathophysiology

Chronic aortic regurgitation

With malcoaptation during diastole, a portion of the left ventricular SV regurgitates back from the aorta into the LV. The subsequent increase in LV end-diastolic volume augments wall stress, resulting in compensatory **eccentric hypertrophy**. Left ventricular volume is increased; however, as compliance is also increased, end-diastolic pressure remains normal.

These adaptations sustain an effective forward SV and cardiac output despite the regurgitation. Whereas diastolic pressure falls in the wake of the regurgitant fraction, systolic pressure is elevated, courtesy of the increased SV, resulting in a wide pulse pressure with characteristic 'bounding pulse' clinical signs. Typically, disease progression is slow and insidious with low morbidity and a long asymptomatic period. However, a proportion of patients will eventually develop severe AR, with subsequent left ventricular dilation, systolic dysfunction, and ultimately heart failure.

Acute aortic regurgitation

In acute AR, a normal ventricular size results in a marked increase in end-diastolic pressure relative to the regurgitant volume. In contrast to chronic AR, the forward SV is impaired, resulting in reduced systolic pressure and a narrow pulse pressure. Indeed, reliance on pulse pressure as an indicator of regurgitation may significantly underestimate the severity of acute AR. The elevated left ventricular diastolic pressure may force early closure of the MV, impeding left ventricular filling; pre-existing impaired diastolic function may exacerbate this decompensation. Coronary ischaemia may develop as a result of reduced diastolic coronary flow, coupled with increased myocardial oxygen demand from elevated end-diastolic pressures and tachycardia. Compensatory tachycardia may preserve cardiac output initially, but eventually cardiogenic shock and pulmonary oedema ensue.

Echocardiographic assessment of aortic regurgitation

Echocardiographic assessment should confirm the diagnosis and severity of AR, examine aortic anatomy and dimensions, evaluate PAPs, and determine right and left ventricular size and function.

2D and M-mode

Use 2D to assess:

- Valve anatomy:
  - Is the valve tri-leaflet?
- Systolic doming:
  - An asymmetric closure line suggests a bicuspid valve
- Commissural fusion (rheumatic heart disease)
- Leaflet mobility, calcification, or thickening
- Vegetations or aortic root abscess (endocarditis)
- LVOT and root anatomy:
  - Annulus, sinuses, and sinotubular junction diameters
- Evidence of dissection
- Evidence of coexistent congenital defects (for example, ventricular septal defect)
- Left ventricular structure and function, specifically chamber size:
  - May help determine acuity—dilation implies chronicity—and prognosis
- The presence or absence of eccentric hypertrophy
- Left ventricular function (impaired function may imply haemodynamically severe AR).

> **Practice point**
>
> Aortic dissection can present as acute severe AR. Aortic dissection involves cleavage and separation of an intimal flap and creation of a false lumen that emanates from an intimal tear. Distal and proximal propagation may

disrupt branch vessels, the aortic valve, and the pericardium, inducing ischaemia, AR, and cardiac tamponade. TTE can afford timely diagnosis, which is critical for survival. A dissection flap may be discernible as a mobile, linear structure, with motion independent of the aortic wall in all aortic views (parasternal, subcostal, and suprasternal). A false lumen may be identifiable by different flow patterns in the true and false lumens under colour Doppler interrogation. Secondary complications should also be ruled out; the aortic root (parasternally), aortic arch and descending aorta (suprasternally), and abdominal aorta (subcostally) should all be measured, the pericardium examined, the LV assessed, and any AR should be quantified. Note that a negative transthoracic exam does not exclude dissection—where there is a high index of suspicion, further imaging with CT or TOE should be considered.

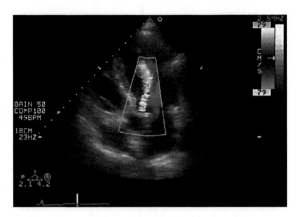

Figure 5.11 [Video 5.5] Apical five-chamber view with a colour Doppler box over the aortic valve and left ventricular outflow tract, demonstrating central aortic regurgitation into the left ventricle. For a colour version of this figure, please see colour plate section.

🎥 *This video is available to watch in the online video appendix.*

© Oxford University Hospitals NHS Foundation Trust 2016, with permission.

Doppler assessment

Colour Doppler

Colour-flow Doppler is a highly sensitive technique for the detection of AR (Figure 5.11 🎥) which enables accurate visualization and qualitative assessment of the regurgitant jet. Colour can be used to detect whether the regurgitant flow is central, eccentric, or commissural, or even if it is through a perforation.

The extent of regurgitant flow into the left ventricular cavity is not a very reliable measure of severity, as many factors influence the colour jet size, including machine settings, jet turbulence, and eccentricity. Colour Doppler is principally a qualitative assessment of severity that is complementary to other assessments.

Vena contracta

The vena contracta (VC) of aortic regurgitant flow is the width of the narrowest portion of colour flow at the level of the aortic valve in the LVOT, immediately below the flow convergence zone, and is an approximation of the regurgitant orifice diameter. Ideally, it

should be assessed in the parasternal long axis view with zoom applied. It is usually a small measurement and thus prone to error with inappropriate gain settings and poor resolution, and it is unreliable in the presence of multiple jets or an irregularly shaped orifice (Figure 5.12) 🎥. Eccentric jets, however, can be accurately assessed if the measurement is made perpendicular to the jet, rather than the LVOT. A VC of <0.3 cm suggests mild AR, and >0.6 cm suggests severe AR.

Jet width as a proportion of left ventricular outflow tract

VC width relative to the LVOT diameter is a useful guide to severity. As with VC, measurement is undertaken in a zoomed parasternal long axis view, but with colour M-mode to maximize spatial and temporal resolution (Figure 5.13).

A jet which occupies <25% of the width suggests mild AR, whereas >65% implies severe AR. Using M-mode, LVOT width is measured in the same axis as the VC, so eccentric jets may result in underestimation of severity. Also, as the jet expands distal to the flow convergence zone, measurement too far into the LVOT will result in overestimation.

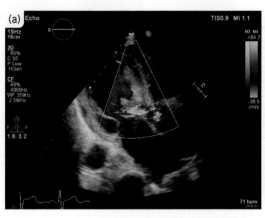 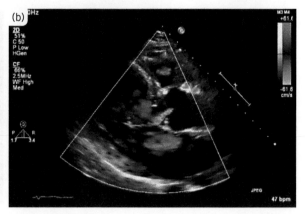

Figure 5.12 (a) [Video 5.6] and 5.12 (b) [Video 5.7] Parasternal long axis view with colour Doppler over the left ventricular outflow tract, demonstrating aortic regurgitation. For a colour version of this figure, please see colour plate section.

● *These videos are available to watch in the online video appendix.*

© Oxford University Hospitals NHS Foundation Trust 2016, with permission.

Pressure half-time and jet deceleration rate

The speed at which the regurgitant velocity decays is proportional to the severity of AR; the pressure between the aorta and ventricle equalizes more rapidly with increasing severity. The $P_{1/2}$ is the time taken for pressure across the valve to fall by 50% and is derived from measurement of the peak velocity and the deceleration slope. In an apical five- or three-chamber view, continuous wave is aligned through the colour-mapped regurgitation jet. Ideally, the Doppler should pass through the regurgitant

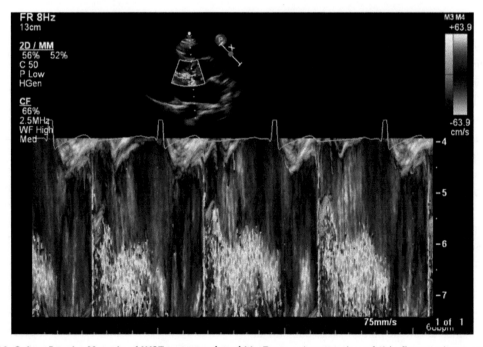

Figure 5.13 Colour Doppler M-mode of LVOT to assess jet width. For a colour version of this figure, please see colour plate section.

© Oxford University Hospitals NHS Foundation Trust 2016, with permission.

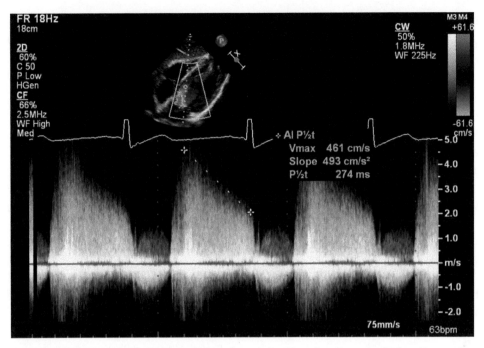

Figure 5.14 **Pressure half-time measurement of continuous-wave Doppler of aortic regurgitation.** For a colour version of this figure, please see colour plate section.

© Oxford University Hospitals NHS Foundation Trust 2016, with permission.

orifice and align along the length of the jet; for eccentric jets, off-axis views may be necessary.

Peak velocity (usually 4–6 m/s) and the slope of the flat portion of the curve should be measured. $P_{1/2}$ will generally correlate inversely with the deceleration slope—the shorter the $P_{1/2}$, the greater the gradient of the slope (Figure 5.14). A $P_{1/2}$ of >500 ms is considered mild, and <200 ms severe. $P_{1/2}$ is probably a more accurate reflection of severity in acute AR. With progressive chronic AR, the LV adapts to accommodate increasingly larger regurgitant volumes. This slows the equalization in pressure and prolongs $P_{1/2}$. The density of the waveform may also communicate severity—as density approaches that of the systolic waveform, severity increases.

Volumetric methods using pulsed Doppler

In AR, the SV at the LVOT exceeds that at MV inflow, assuming there is no significant MR. Therefore, the volume of AR equals LVOT SV ($LVOT_{SV}$) minus MV SV (MV_{SV}), where:

$$LVOT_{SV} = CSA_{LVOT} \times VTI_{LVOT}$$

$$MV_{SV} = CSA_{MV} \times VTI_{MV}$$

Pulsed-wave Doppler is used to measure VTI, and zoomed images with the valves open used to measure the diameters.

$$CSA_{LVOT} = \pi \times (LVOT\ diameter/2)^2$$

$$CSA_{MV} = \pi \times (MV\ diameter/2)^2$$

The calculations are prone to error and often impractical for rapid assessments of severity.

Supporting evidence for evaluating aortic regurgitation

Continuous-wave Doppler of aortic regurgitation velocity

The intensity of the regurgitant signal seen on continuous-wave spectral display in apical three- or five-chamber views reflects the volume of regurgitation through the aortic valve. Equalization of density with forward flow indicates severe AR.

Diastolic flow reversal

Pulsed-wave Doppler interrogation of the upper descending aorta (from a suprasternal view) may detect brief (early) reversal of diastolic aortic flow, even in normal individuals. However, with increasing severity, flow reversal occupies a greater period of diastole and diastolic flow velocities increase. Pandiastolic flow reversal indicates at least moderate regurgitation. A VTI of >15 cm is considered to be consistent with severe AR. Colour M-mode can also be helpful to evaluate flow direction (Figure 5.15).

Combined echo assessment of aortic regurgitation

Table 5.5 shows the direct and indirect echo features of AR and how they influence grading the severity.

Aortic regurgitation in critical care

Mild to moderate AR is commonly encountered on the ICU and is generally well tolerated.

AR as a primary reason for admission to the ICU is likely to be as a result of aortic valve endocarditis or aortic dissection and will therefore usually be acute. In this setting, echocardiography (Figure 5.16 🎦) will demonstrate:

- A hyperdynamic, non-dilated LV
- Premature MV closure, evidenced by MV fluttering on M-mode in the PLAX view
- AR on colour Doppler.

Pharmacological support for severe acute AR is limited since:

- Vasopressors may increase the degree of AR
- Inotropes increase myocardial oxygen demand and reduce diastolic and therefore coronary filling time, increasing the risk of coronary ischaemia, which is already raised by the regurgitant fraction
- Sedative drugs almost universally have a directly negative inotropic effect on the myocardium and may increase the time for regurgitation during diastole by inducing bradycardia.

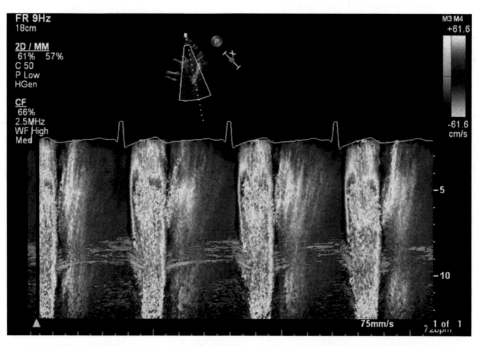

Figure 5.15 Colour M-mode of flow in the descending thoracic aorta from a suprasternal position. Flow is retrograde (red) for the whole of diastole due to severe AR. For a colour version of this figure, please see colour plate section.
© Oxford University Hospitals NHS Foundation Trust 2016, with permission.

Practice point

Make a diagnosis using echocardiography guided by history and clinical examination.

- Use sedative drugs with limited direct effect on the myocardium; avoid propofol.
- Where essential to maintain cardiovascular integrity, use low doses of vasopressors and inotropes; higher doses will result in cardiovascular collapse.
- Offset and treat bradycardia of <80 bpm.
- Early discussion with surgical colleagues since surgical management is the only definitive treatment option.

Occasionally, patients will present to critical care with coexisting chronic severe AR.

Echocardiographic findings depend on the chronicity of the valve lesion and therefore will demonstrate echocardiographic findings along a spectrum from those of acute AR to a dilated and impaired ventricle due to prolonged exposure to high regurgitant volumes. Severe chronic AR with evidence of subsequent left ventricular dilatation and dysfunction is likely to

precipitate cardiovascular collapse in conjunction with major systemic illness such as haemorrhage or sepsis.

Practice point

Make an early diagnosis using echocardiography guided by history and clinical examination.

- The echocardiographic finding of severe chronic AR with subsequent left ventricular dilatation and dysfunction should be included in decision-making about the usefulness of further multi-organ support in the context of the patient's best interests.
- Where it is deemed appropriate to continue with multi-organ support, the principles of cardiovascular management are as for acute AR.
- Maintain a stable moderate SVR, and avoid bradycardias from whatever cause.

Mitral regurgitation

The MV is the most anatomically and physiologically complex of all the cardiac valves. Two leaflets, set within a saddle-shaped annulus, open in diastole to

Table 5.5 The direct and indirect echo features of AR and how they influence grading the severity

Quantitative parameters	Mild	Moderate	Severe
Vena contracta width (cm)	<0.3		>0.6
Jet width/LVOT diameter (%)	<25		≥65
Regurgitant volume (mL)	≤30	31–59	≥60
Regurgitant fraction (%)	≤30	31–49	≥50
Regurgitant orifice area (cm²)	≤0.10	0.11–0.29	≥0.30
$P_{1/2}$ (ms)	>500		<20
End-diastolic velocity (upper DAo) (cm/s)			≥20
Supportive features			
Diastolic flow reversal in descending aorta	Minimal	Intermediate features between mild and severe	Holodiastolic
Left ventricular appearance	Normal		Dilatation ± hypertrophy

Data from *Echocardiography: guidelines for Valve and Chamber Quantification*. British Society of Echocardiography, London, 2012 http://www.bsecho.org/media/40506/chamber-final-2011_2_.pdf

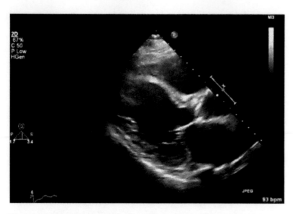

Figure 5.16 [Video 5.8] A patient with acute severe aortic regurgitation secondary to aortic valve endocarditis.

🔘 *This video is available to watch in the online video appendix.*
© Oxford University Hospitals NHS Foundation Trust 2016, with permission.

allow unobstructed flow through a large orifice, from the low-pressure LA into the LV. During systole, an intricate scaffolding of chordae attached to two specialized areas of ventricular papillary muscle (PM) anchor the leaflets to prevent leaflet prolapse and regurgitation from the high-pressure LV to the low-pressure LA.

MV closure is an active process—a 'closing force' generated in systole acts against the under-surface of the leaflets, 'forcing' them to coapt, counteracting the 'tethering' force of the PM/chordae structure. Proper function of the MV then depends on normal morphology, geometry, and coordination of all these components.

Primary (organic) mitral regurgitation

In primary MR, 'it is the abnormal valve that makes the heart sick'. The LV becomes chronically volume-overloaded and the EF will increase, though a significant proportion of the EF may be retrograde into the LA; in this way, a 'normal' EF implies significant left ventricular impairment. Over time, the LV and LA dilate. Higher wall stress ensues, resulting in further chamber (and mitral annular) dilatation, with potential exacerbation of MR. Progressive MR leads to contractile dysfunction and left ventricular failure. Ultimately, and in common with secondary MR, raised left atrial pressure leads to elevated pulmonary venous pressure and PHT.

Degenerative (myxomatous) MR is the most common cause of MR in the Western world. Degenerative changes may result in MR despite normal leaflet motion, due to annular calcification and dilatation or leaflet calcification and thickenin, or via excessive motion as in MV leaflet prolapse (MVP) or flail sections. MVP—bulging of leaflets >2 mm beyond the mitral annular plane in systole—is the most common presentation of degenerative MR. Flail stipulates eversion of a leaflet segment into the LA; it usually follows chordal rupture, resulting in severe MR.

Less commonly, **infective endocarditis** (IE) may cause MR through leaflet malcoaptation secondary to valvular vegetations, chordal rupture, paravalvular abscess, or leaflet aneurysm, or following leaflet perforation. **Rheumatic, inflammatory, and iatrogenic** causes of MR present relatively infrequently.

Secondary (functional) mitral regurgitation

The terms **functional** and **ischaemic** MR (IMR) are often used interchangeably to describe **secondary** MR—that is, MR without MV leaflet abnormalities. Adverse local or global left ventricular remodelling—of either ischaemic or non-ischaemic origin—induces posterolateral PM displacement and annular dilatation. Tethering of the MV leaflets by the displaced PM results in systolic restriction of MV leaflet motion and malcoaptation (Figure 5.17).

Acute mitral regurgitation

Acute native valve MR can be structural or functional, as shown in Table 5.6. Mechanisms include the development of a flail segment from either ruptured papillary muscle (acute MI or trauma) or chordae tendinae (myxomatous disease, endocarditis, rheumatic mitral valve disease, or trauma), leaflet rupture (endocarditis), or acute on chronic (dynamic) MR (see later text).

The haemodynamics of acute MR reflect the lack of adaptation of the LA and LV to the MR. The sudden increase in volume into the non-compliant LA causes elevated left atrial pressure and subsequently pulmonary oedema. As the LV is not dilated, the majority of blood is regurgitated, and forward flow is compromised. The presentation can be dramatic, with rapid progression to cardiogenic shock, exacerbated by

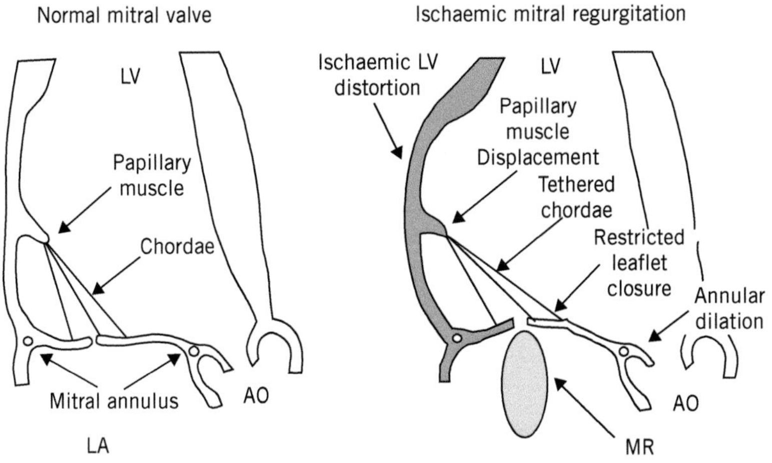

Normal mitral valve   Ischaemic mitral regurgitation

Figure 5.17 Demonstration of how changes in left ventricular geometry lead to mitral regurgitation.
Reprinted from *Progress in Cardiovascular Diseases*, 57, 1, Zeng X, Tan TC, Dudzinski DM, Hung J, 'Echocardiography of the mitral valve', pp. 55–73, Copyright 2014, with permission from Elsevier

increased peripheral resistance; MR worsens, cardiac output falls, and cardiovascular collapse ensues.

Echocardiographic assessment of mitral regurgitation

Echocardiographic assessment should focus on determination of the mechanism and acuity of MR. Use of 2D in all four standard transthoracic views enables detailed examination of the diseased valve and chambers, and the application of Doppler methods greatly assists in the quantification of severity.

2D and M-mode

2D and M-mode should be used to assess the structure of the valve and subvalvular apparatus. Key elements the examination should aim to identify include:

- Leaflet appearance:
  - Look for evidence of myxomatous degeneration, rheumatic valve disease, thickening, or calcification
- Leaflet mobility:
  - Prolapse or flail; restricted mobility in systole and diastole; systolic tethering or 'tenting'
- Leaflet structural integrity:
  - Perforations
- Leaflet coaptation integrity

- Leaflet vegetation presence:
  - Location, mobility, dimensions
- Chordae tendinae appearance:
  - Signs of degeneration/calcification; rupture
- PM integrity
- Annular size
- Left atrial enlargement as a marker of chronicity
- Left ventricular size, shape, and function:
  - Dimensions, systolic function, presence of regional wall motion abnormalities
- Right heart assessment:
  - Right ventricular function, evidence of PHT.

Doppler assessment

Quantification of MR severity using Doppler is arguably one of the most challenging tasks in echocardiography. It relies on assessment of the regurgitant jet, which has three elements: the proximal flow convergence zone or proximal isovelocity surface area (PISA), the VC, and the distal jet. The proximal flow convergence zone occurs 'upstream' of the regurgitant orifice. The VC represents the narrowest point at the leaflets or just distal to the leaflets; it is the effective regurgitant orifice area (EROA) defined by flow, and not the anatomic orifice area defined by the anatomy. The distal regurgitant jet represents the final flow as it enters the LA.

Table 5.6 Classification of MR

	Primary (organic)	Secondary (functional)
Acute	Flail MV leaflet Ruptured PM (trauma, infarction) Ruptured chordae tendinae Endocarditis Leaflet perforation	Acute local or global ischaemia or MI Ventricular dyssynchrony New-onset left bundle branch block Temporary right ventricular pacing Acute LVOT obstruction Hypertrophic cardiomyopathy Takotsubo's/apical ballooning syndrome Hypovolaemia
Chronic	Degenerative (myxomatous) Carpentier I (annulus and/or leaflet calcification) Carpentier II (MVP, flail MV leaflet (ruptured chordae tendinae)) Endocarditis Leaflet malcoaptation (vegetations, abscess) Rheumatic Congenital	Chronic ischaemic MR (CIMR) Non-ischaemic cardiomyopathy (left ventricular dilatation and/or systolic dysfunction) Chronic right ventricular pacing

Adapted from Dudzinski DM and Hung J, 'Echocardiographic assessment of ischemic mitral regurgitation', *Cardiovascular Ultrasound*, 2014 Nov 21;12:46. © Dudzinski and Hung; licensee BioMed Central Ltd. 2014 https://cardiovascularultrasound.biomedcentral.com/articles/10.1186/1476-7120-12-46. This article is published under license to BioMed Central Ltd. This is an Open Access article distributed under the terms of the Creative Commons Attribution License (http://creativecommons.org/licenses/by/4.0), which permits unrestricted use, distribution, and reproduction in any medium, provided the original work is properly credited. The Creative Commons Public Domain Dedication waiver (http://creativecommons.org/publicdomain/zero/1.0/) applies to the data made available in this article, unless otherwise stated.

Colour Doppler jet area

Colour Doppler interrogation over the LA enables the simplest assessment of the regurgitant jet—essentially, how big the regurgitant jet is relative to the size of the LA. Best assessed in an apical four-chamber view, the jet area (JA) is determined as the maximum JA to left atrial area ratio where the left atrial area is measured in the same frame as the maximum JA, as shown in Figure 5.18 . The maximal JA should be measured in multiple views and the average taken.

Imaging in multiple views also allows assessment of:

- Jet direction (eccentricity of a jet often signifies disease of the contralateral leaflet)
- Mechanism of regurgitation (central, through leaflet perforation, systolic anterior motion (SAM), etc.)
- Number of jets.

The size of the jet only provides a guide to severity and should be correlated with additional parameters.

Potential pitfalls include:

- Incorrect settings: gain—lower sampling limit may overestimate severity
- Jet eccentricity: jets may flatten out against the atrial wall, leading to under-estimation
- Direction of jet flow: jets which traverse the imaging plane may be under-estimated
- Entrainment of blood adjacent to the jet may result in overestimation.

Vena contracta

Measurement of the VC diameter allows estimation of the EROA. Ideally, it should be assessed in views orthogonal to the coaptation plane, such as the PLAX or apical four-chamber, to avoid overestimation. As it is a small measure, it is prone to error; as a result of inappropriate gain settings and poor resolution, small absolute errors in measurement translate into proportionally large inaccuracies. Other limitations include the under-estimation of MR in the presence of multiple jets and poor performance in the presence of an irregularly shaped orifice.

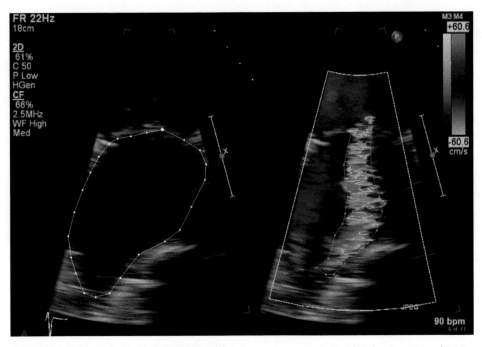

Figure 5.18 [Video 5.9] Estimation of mitral regurgitation jet size, compared to left atrial size from the apical four-chamber position. For a colour version of this figure, please see colour plate section.

🔵 *This video is available to watch in the online video appendix.*

© Oxford University Hospitals NHS Foundation Trust 2016, with permission.

PISA assessment

The PISA method is based on the fluid dynamics principle that as flow approaches a finite circular orifice, it forms concentric hemispheric shells with a gradually decreasing surface area and an increasing velocity. In relation to MR, the PISA is the hemispheric region that forms proximal to the MV leaflets on the left ventricular side, and the finite orifice is the regurgitant orifice at the level of the leaflets.

Assuming a hemispheric shape for the isovelocity shells, then the MR flow rate equals the product of the surface area and the shell's aliasing velocity. The surface area of the shell equals $2\pi r^2$ where r is the radius of the hemispheric shell. The EROA can be derived using the following formula:

$$EROA = \frac{(PISA\ area \times Aliasing\ velocity)}{MR\ peak\ velocity}$$

Magnifying the PISA region with sector and depth optimized for colour resolution and shifting the baseline of the Nyquist limit in the direction of flow to 20–40 cm/

s will provide the optimal conditions for accurate and reproducible PISA estimations (Figure 5.19).

An EROA of <0.2 is mild, and ≥0.4 is severe. Given the complexity, this technique is rarely practicable in critically ill patients.

Volumetric assessment using pulsed Doppler

The difference between chamber inflow and outflow volumes (that is SV) represents the regurgitant volume. The MR volume (MR_{vol}) is typically calculated as MV inflow minus aortic outflow. The SV across any valve can be calculated by multiplying the cross-sectional area by flow at that point, as used in the continuity equation.

The MV annulus diameter is measured in the apical four-chamber view. For aortic outflow, the diameter of the LVOT is measured in the parasternal long axis position.

$$SV_{MV} = CSA_{MV} \times VTI_{MV}$$

$$SV_{LVOT} = CSA_{LVOT} \times VTI_{LVOT}, \text{ and}$$

$$MR_{vol} = SV_{MV} - SV_{LVOT}$$

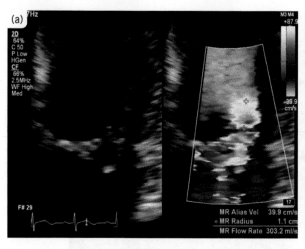

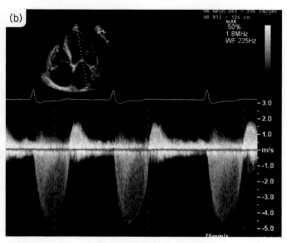

Figure 5.19 (a) and (b) **Quantification of mitral regurgitation.** For a colour version of Figure 5.19 (a), please see colour plate section.

© Oxford University Hospitals NHS Foundation Trust 2016, with permission.

The MR fraction may then be calculated as:

$$RF = (MR_{vol} / MV_{SV}) \times 100$$

The sheer number of measurements and assumptions involved makes this technique prone to variability; like PISA, in the acute setting, this technique may prove cumbersome.

Supporting evidence for evaluating mitral regurgitation

Pulmonary venous inflow pattern

The pattern of **pulmonary venous inflow** varies with MR severity. Inflow occurs during both systole and diastole; the systolic (S) wave is normally slightly larger than the diastolic (D) wave. Pulmonary veins are sampled in the apical four-chamber view, with the sample placed 1 cm into the vein. With increasing MR severity, the S wave is correspondingly dampened, decreasing below the D wave and ultimately reversing (Figure 5.20).

Continuous-wave Doppler of the mitral regurgitation velocity

Aligning continuous-wave Doppler with the MR jet in the apical four-chamber view provides a qualitative assessment of the regurgitant volume. The intensity—and completeness—of the continuous-wave Doppler signal correlates with MR severity. In very severe MR, rapid equilibration of the LV–LA pressure gradient results not only in reduced signal velocity, but also in an altered trace morphology—the characteristic parabolic continuous wave MR signal transforms into a 'V' shape.

Other supportive features

Raised right ventricular systolic pressures may reflect significant regurgitation into the pulmonary venous system. Raised mitral inflow velocity (as evidenced by increased E wave velocity) also suggests significant MR in the absence of MS. Increased left atrial and left ventricular chamber sizes are associated with long-standing MR.

Combined echo assessment of mitral regurgitation

Table 5.7 shows the direct and indirect echo features of MR and how they influence grading the severity.

Dynamic mitral regurgitation in critical illness

Dynamic variation in the severity of MR can be seen in critical illness, whatever the underlying cause of the regurgitation.

Factors exacerbating MR: these factors reduce overall left ventricular work and increase left ventricular afterload:

- Tachycardia or arrhythmias
- High SVR

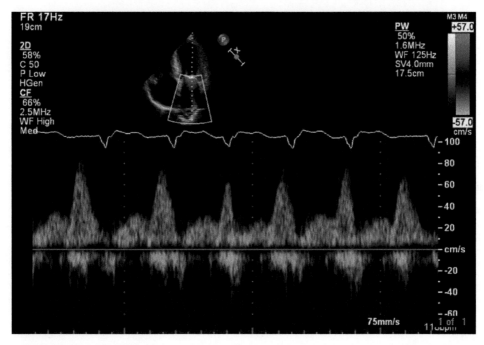

Figure 5.20 Pulsed Doppler of the right upper pulmonary vein from the apical four-chamber position—abnormal blunting of the systolic waveform is demonstrated.

© Oxford University Hospitals NHS Foundation Trust 2016, with permission.

- Maldistributive shock
- Transient myocardial ischaemia: reversibly worsens left ventricular geometry and function
- Fluid loading
- Any increase in myocardial oxygen demand, for example in drug overdose or sepsis.

Factors reducing the severity of MR: these factors tend to reduce overall left ventricular workload and level off afterload:

- Vasodilatation
- Haemofiltration
- Negatively inotropic sedative drugs
- Invasive and non-invasive ventilation: reduce left ventricular loading by opposing right ventricular outflow.

The haemodynamic variability that characterizes MR in critical care may make accurate assessment difficult. For example, patients may have minimal MR when sedated and ventilated but have a significant regurgitant fraction when these factors are altered. Echocardiography performed under different loading conditions is therefore key to severity assessment; this is particularly relevant in patients who are failing to wean from mechanical ventilation when echo assessment should be repeated during an SBT.

Where MR is thought to be significantly contributing to cardiovascular failure or failure to wean, the following elements of circulation should be optimized:

- Minimize fluid loading
- Avoid tachycardia
- Encourage sinus rhythm
- Vasodilate
- Avoid high SVR
- Use non-invasive or invasive ventilation to off-load the ventricle and allow a return of haemodynamic balance.

In the setting of PM rupture/flail MV leaflet, these measures will be inadequate and emergency surgical referral is indicated. Intubation and ventilation are hazardous in this setting without immediate access to

Table 5.7 Direct and indirect echo features of MR and how they influence grading the severity

Quantitative parameters	Mild	Moderate	Severe
VC width (cm)	<0.3		≥0.7
PISA radius CM (Nyquist 40 cm/s)	<0.4		>1.0
Regurgitant volume (mL)	≤30	31–59	≥60
Regurgitant fraction (%)	≤30	31–49	≥50
Regurgitant orifice area (cm²)	<0.20	0.21–0.39	≥0.40
MV inflow(VTI)/LVOT(VTI)			>1.4
Supportive features			
Pulmonary venous flow	Systolic dominant	Intermediate features between mild and severe	Diastolic dominant
E/A ratio	A wave dominant		E wave dominant (>1.2 m/s)
Continuous-wave Doppler signal appearance	Soft density parabolic arc		Dense, triangular jet
Left atrial and left ventricular appearance			Dilated LA and LV

Data from Echocardiography: guidelines for Valve and Chamber Quantification. British Society of Echocardiography, London, 2012 http://www.bsecho.org/media/40506/chamber-final-2011_2_.pdf.

cardiopulmonary bypass but may be the only bridge to theatre where the valve is acutely and catastrophically disrupted. Induction of anaesthesia should be slow and opiate- and benzodiazepine-based, to avoid changes in SVR and left ventricular function.

> **Practice point**
>
> The interplay between the function and geometry of the LV and the anatomy of the MV, along with preload, afterload, and heart rate, all influence the degree of MR. Assessment of lesion severity must take into account the prevailing haemodynamic situation, and, if necessary, modification of afterload with dynamic assessment of MV function should be undertaken.

Diagnosing and managing infective endocarditis

Definition

Infective endocarditis (IE) is infection of the abnormal valve endothelium by bacteria, leading to clusters of fibrin, platelets, leucocytes, and bacteria which form vegetations and inflammation, then valve destruction and abscess formation.

IE can be classified in many ways, but a practical system defines IE as:

- Native or prosthetic valve
- Left- or right-sided infection
- Device-related—involving pacemaker or catheter
- Community-acquired
- Relapsing
- Culture-negative.

Overall mortality from IE remains high at around 25% despite medical and surgical management.

Aetiology

Although IE can occur on normal native valves, it is more commonly seen in patients with an underlying valve or endothelial pathology. Certain features predispose patients to a higher risk of endocarditis and include:

- Prosthetic valves of any form
- Previously treated IE
- Complex congenital heart disease
- Left-to-right intracardiac shunts.

Factors that increase the risk of acquiring IE are:

- Intravenous drug use
- Severe dental disease
- Diabetes
- Immunosuppression
- Renal failure
- Pregnancy
- Central venous catheter use.

The majority of cases are caused by bacterial pathogens, and most of these are Gram-positive cocci such as *Staphylococcus aureus* and *epidermidis*, *Streptococcus*, and *Enterococcus*. Rarer cases with Gram-negative pathogens do occur; fungal IE is usually only seen in the severely immunocompromised.

The historical 'subacute' bacterial endocarditis is becoming rare, and the majority of cases are acute with a marked increase in IE due to *S. aureus* which causes aggressive, rapidly enlarging, and destructive vegetations, with a high embolic risk and high mortality. Cases of IE in intravenous drug users and patients with indwelling vascular access catheters or pacemakers are also increasing.

Diagnostic criteria

If IE is suspected, then diagnosis requires integration of clinical, microbiological, and echocardiographic data in that order. The most important test in suspected IE is multiple blood cultures before antibiotic administration.

A definite diagnosis can be made using the modified Duke criteria (Table 5.8) which requires one of the following:

- Two major criteria present
- One major and three minor criteria
- Five minor criteria.

In suspected cases, prompt microbiological evaluation with cultures and imaging assessment with TTE is needed.

Table 5.8 Modified Duke criteria for the clinical diagnosis of infective endocarditis

Major criteria	Minor criteria
Culture of a typical IE organism from two separate samples	Predisposing factor
Vegetation on echocardiography	Fever
Abscess identified	Evidence of embolic phenomena
Prosthetic valve dehiscence	Immune-mediated phenomena
New valvular regurgitation	Atypical cultures

Reproduced from JS Li, Sexton, D.J., Mick N.*et al.*, 'Proposed Modifications to the Duke Criteria for the Diagnosis of Infective Endocarditis', *Clinical Infectious Diseases*, 2000, 30, 4, pp. 633–638, by permission of Infectious Diseases Society of America.

Assessment using transthoracic echo

TTE has a sensitivity of only 50–60% for confirming IE, so a negative study does not fully exclude this pathology. False positives can occur if other lesions, such as ruptured chordae, fibroelastoma, or thickened nodules, are misinterpreted as vegetations.

The typical features of vegetations include:

- Texture similar to the myocardium and not echo-bright
- 'Upstream' side of valve, that is the left atrial side of the MV (Figure 5.21)
- Oscillating motion and prolapse into upstream chamber
- Lobulated shape
- Attached to prosthetic material if present.

Suspected vegetations should be measured and the maximum size reported, along with the degree of mobility, as these influence the potential embolic risk. Valve destruction usually leads to regurgitation, although large vegetations can obstruct flow and lead to stenosis. The mechanism of regurgitation should be evaluated and can be due to:

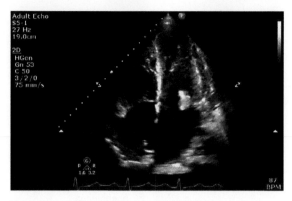

Figure 5.21 [Video 5.10] A large vegetation on the posterior leaflet of the mitral valve.
This video is available to watch in the online video appendix.
© Oxford University Hospitals NHS Foundation Trust 2016, with permission.

- Leaflet perforation
- Leaflet destruction and flail portion
- Paravalvular regurgitation due to abscess erosion and dehiscence.

When to request a transoesophageal echo?

All patients with suspected IE should undergo assessment with TTE first. If the clinical suspicion is high and the TTE is non-confirmatory, then a TOE is required.

A TOE should also be performed in the following situations:

- Confirmed IE on TTE—to evaluate the lesion in more detail and identify complications
- Prosthetic valve endocarditis
- New complications such as heart block or embolic event
- Presence of intracardiac prosthetic material such as a pacemaker
- Initial negative TOE, but high clinical suspicion—repeat after 7 days.

Management

Treatment of IE involves prolonged and tailored antimicrobial therapy and vigilant monitoring for complications. Empirical therapy can be commenced in acutely unwell patients as long as blood cultures have been performed; in more stable patients, awaiting microbiology information is helpful.

Prolonged antimicrobial therapy for 2–6 weeks, depending on the organism and patient factors, is needed in all cases and may be sufficient to cure the infection. Careful monitoring of progress and development of side effects from high-dose antimicrobials is essential.

Surgery for infective endocarditis

Early surgery should be considered in patients with the following features:

- Progressive heart failure despite medical therapy
- Uncontrolled infection—abscess formation or enlarging vegetation (Figure 5.22)
- Staphylococcal infection
- Fungal infection—large vegetations occur
- Persistent fever
- Recurrent embolic events despite medical therapy
- Prosthetic valve dehiscence.

Prosthetic valve endocarditis almost always requires surgical treatment. Traditional management of all forms of IE recommended prolonged medical therapy and delayed surgery, but current evidence and guidelines suggest a low threshold for early surgery. Discussion and transfer to a cardiac surgical centre are appropriate in many cases.

Complications

The potential complications of IE are numerous, and the majority relate to the presence of highly embolic infection material within the bloodstream.

Intracardiac complications include:

- Heart failure due to severe valvular regurgitation
- Abscess or fistula formation
- Aortic dissection
- Coronary embolization and MI.

Extracardiac manifestations include:

- Stroke due to cerebral embolism
- Intracerebral haemorrhage due to rupture of a mycotic aneurysm

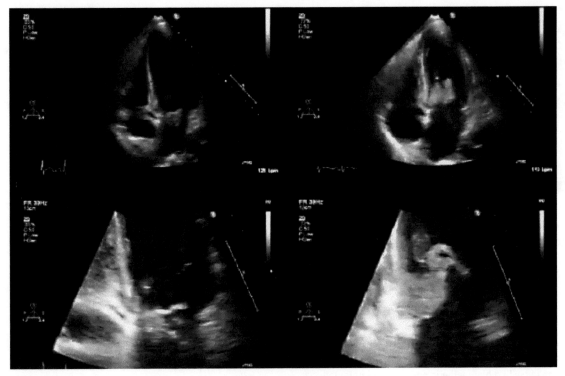

Figure 5.22 [Video 5.11] Progressive increase in vegetation size despite antibiotic therapy in a patient with *S. aureus* native mitral valve endocarditis presenting with a stroke.

This video is available to watch in the online video appendix.

© Oxford University Hospitals NHS Foundation Trust 2016, with permission.

- Peripheral ischaemia from emboli
- Renal infarction
- Osteomyelitis
- Discitis
- Ototoxicity from aminoglycosides
- Nephrotoxicity from antimicrobials
- Allergic reactions
- Vascular access complications.

CASE STUDY

Endocarditis in critical care

A 42-year-old male living in a local hostel was admitted with acute confusion and delirium. Aggression and disorientation on arrival at A&E warranted sedation to allow assessment but provoked circulatory collapse with hypotension, tachycardia, and hypoxia.

An initial diagnosis of acute meningo-encephalitis was made, and after three sets of peripheral blood cultures were taken, broad-spectrum antibiotics were administered. The patient was paralysed, intubated, ventilated, and transferred to critical care for haemodynamic support. A rapidly developing, widespread rash was noted, along with suspected infective arthritis of the right wrist.

After 48 hours of intensive support with fluids, vasopressors, and antibiotics, the patient was stable enough for extubation. He reported pain and swelling in the right hand 2 days prior to admission and admitted to intravenous drug use. Cultures taken on admission confirmed *S. aureus*, and a TTE identified a 16-mm vegetation on a bicuspid aortic valve with moderate AR (Figure 5.23 ●).

Resolution of bacteraemia and fever occurred over the following 3 days, and the patient was transferred to the cardiology department. On day 10, the patient experienced acute left arm and leg weakness whilst showering, and a CT brain identified a new cerebral infarction but no haemorrhage. Urgent TOE demonstrated an increase in vegetation

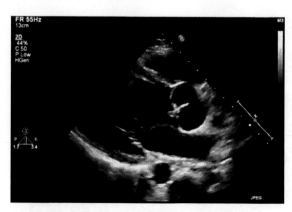

Figure 5.23 [Video 5.12] Infective endocarditis of a bicuspid aortic valve with leaflet perforation and a vegetation evident.

🔘 *This video is available to watch in the online video appendix.*
© Oxford University Hospitals NHS Foundation Trust 2016, with permission.

size, severe regurgitation due to leaflet destruction, and early abscess formation. Immediate cardiac surgery was undertaken with a bioprosthetic aortic valve implanted.

Six weeks later, the patient had recovered and completed antibiotic therapy and was discharged from hospital. Three months later, he was found unconscious in septi-caemic shock with recurrent *S. aureus* infection of the prosthetic valve due to self-inoculation during intravenous drug administration. Prosthetic valve dehiscence and free regurgitation provoked cardiogenic shock and death before surgery could be attempted.

Multiple choice questions

1. When assessing aortic stenosis:
   A The continuity equation is affected by flow
   B In the presence of severe aortic regurgitation, the peak velocity will be under-estimated
   C Peak aortic velocity is measured using continuous-wave Doppler beyond the aortic valve
   D Dobutamine stress echocardiography is contraindicated
   E An interventricular septal thickness in diastole of 1.1 cm is normal

2. The following are true of mitral stenosis:
   A Systolic dysfunction is infrequently associated
   B Mitral valve planimetry is affected by heart rate
   C The mean gradient should be calculated with pulsed-wave Doppler across the mitral valve
   D A pressure half-time of 170 ms signifies moderate mitral stenosis
   E Beta blockers can be used

3. The following findings are consistent with severe aortic regurgitation:
   A Pressure half-time ($P_{1/2}$) of 250 ms
   B Premature mitral valve closure
   C Narrow pulse pressure
   D Peak trans-aortic pressure gradient of 85 mmHg by Bernoulli equation
   E Descending aorta velocity time integral of 13 s

4. Regarding mitral regurgitation in critical care:
   A An aortic balloon pump is contraindicated
   B Dobutamine may improve mitral regurgitation
   C Positive pressure ventilation is contraindicated
   D A triangular-shaped continuous wave trace is consistent with a sustained LV–LA pressure gradient
   E PISA assessment is always indicated

5. Echocardiographic findings in infective endocarditis typically include:
   A Dense, bright, immobile lesions attached to ventricular endothelium
   B Progressive valve stenosis and obstruction
   C Pericardial effusion
   D Small, thin, strand like structures on the tips of the aortic valve
   E Abscess formation and fistula formation

For answers to multiple choice questions, please see 'Appendix 1: Answers to multiple choice questions', p. 171.

Further reading

Bhattacharyya S, Khattar R, Chahal N, Senior R. Dynamic mitral regurgitation: review of evidence base, assessment and implications for clinical management. *Cardiol Rev* 2015; **23**: 142–7 [Description of mechanisms of mitral regurgitation and implications for management].

Carabello B. The current therapy for mitral regurgitation. *J Am Coll Cardiol* 2008; **52**: 319–26 [Management of acute and chronic mitral regurgitation].

Newton J, Sabharwal N, Myerson S, *et al. Valvular Heart Disease* (Oxford Specialist Handbooks in Cardiology). Oxford University Press, Oxford, 2011 [Handbook on the assessment and management of valvular heart disease, including endocarditis].

Otto CM, Prendergast B. Aortic-valve stenosis—from patients at risk to severe valve obstruction. *N Engl J Med* 2014; **371**: 744–56 [A review of contemporary assessment and management of aortic stenosis].

Wunderlich NC, Beigel R, Siegel RJ. Management of mitral stenosis using 2D and 3D echo-Doppler imaging. *JACC Cardiovasc Imaging* 2013; **6**: 1191–205 [Detailed description of the echo assessment of mitral stenosis].

6

The pericardium

The haemodynamic effects of pericardial disease in the critically ill may be rapidly catastrophic. Comprehensive assessment of the unstable circulation should therefore include the pericardium and its contents. Accurate assessment of tamponade in the critically unwell patient also requires specialist knowledge of the effects of mechanical ventilation on the interplay between the left and right ventricles, a physiological relationship referred to as 'ventricular interdependence'.

Anatomy and physiology

Pericardial anatomy

The pericardium is composed of an inner serous pericardium covering the heart (visceral aspect) and reflecting over the inside of the fibrous pericardium (parietal aspect). The fibrous pericardium forms a thick, outer supportive layer which is suspended from the sternum by the sternopericardial ligaments and from ligamentous attachments to the anterior surface of cervical and upper thoracic vertebrae. The fibrous pericardium is continuous with the central tendon of the diaphragm, the pre-tracheal fascia, and the adventitia of the aorta and pulmonary arteries. These attachments allow the heart to be supported but to move freely inside the thoracic cavity with each cardiac cycle.

Figures 6.1 and 6.2 demonstrate these reflections and attachments.

In health, the space between the fibrous and serous pericardium contains around 50 mL of lubricating fluid at a resting pressure approximately equal to the interpleural pressure. During tidal breathing in an unventilated subject, this resting pressure falls a few centimetres below zero with inspiration, rising to a small positive pressure with expiration.

The fibrous pericardium may become thickened through disease. A thickened, but smooth, appearance is characteristic of acute inflammatory processes, whereas irregular thickening suggests a chronic inflammatory process or post-surgical reaction. Rarely, the pericardium becomes thick and irregular due to calcification from a chronic infiltrative or haemorrhagic process. A thickened, poorly compliant pericardium is a feature of constrictive pericarditis. Although clinically significant, thickening is rare; its diagnosis and accurate quantification are complex and has only recently begun to be understood. As such, these patients need specialist input, particularly when intercurrent critical illness occurs.

Pericardial effusions

A normal volume of pericardial fluid causes partial separation of the fibrous and serous pericardium during the cardiac cycle. This can be seen on echo as an echo-free space in the pericardial position which is <5 mm in depth during diastole.

Greater than 5-mm separation of the fibrous and serous pericardium is abnormal and represents accumulation of pericardial fluid.

This finding should prompt two thought processes:

1. What is the accumulated fluid?
2. What is the current haemodynamic consequence?

Table 6.1 illustrates the common causes of accumulated pericardial fluid in the critically ill. Thinking about the probable cause is important for two reasons.

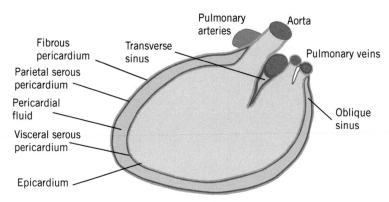

Figure 6.1 Pericardial layers and reflections.

Firstly, by addressing causation, we can think about the likelihood and prevention of recurrence, and secondly drainage of the fluid may be relevant not simply because of circulatory compromise, but also for diagnostic purposes, for example where the accumulated fluid is pus.

Understanding the physiology of cardiac tamponade

As fluid accumulates, the pericardial pressure (PP) begins to rise. If this occurs slowly, then there can be considerable accommodation by stretch of pericardial fibres and the resulting increase in PP is slow.

The effect of pericardial anatomy on cardiac function

Ventricular interdependence is a physiological consequence of the anatomy of the pericardium; since all four cardiac chambers are contained by the fibrous pericardium, a rise in the volume of one chamber will have an impact on the chambers around it. Since the ventricles are larger than the atria, this effect is most potently seen in the filling relationship between the two ventricles, but it also occurs to a certain degree between the ventricles and the atria.

Atrioventricular interdependence

Atrioventricular interdependence (AVI) in health adds to the efficiency of cardiac function. Ventricular systole

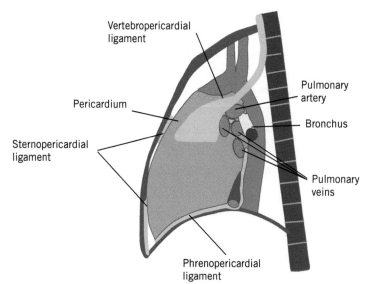

Figure 6.2 Ligamentous attachments of the fibrous pericardium.

Table 6.1 Causes of pericardial fluid accumulation

Category	Pathology	Approximate incidence (%)
Trauma/surgery	Cardiac surgery Intravascular procedures Trauma	20
Medical	Malignant diseases	50
	Uraemia Idiopathic pericarditis	10
	Infectious diseases Anticoagulation or thrombolysis	5
	Connective tissue diseases Renal failure Dressler's syndrome Radiation therapy Renal failure Hypothyroidism Left ventricular pseudoaneurysm	1–5

allows and encourages atrial filling by pulling the atrio-ventricular annulus longitudinally towards the apex and creating space within the pericardium for the atria to passively fill. When the PP is elevated, atrial filling is even more dependent on this process since passive filling is opposed by the raised PP.

Knowledge of this process allows us to see the exaggerated effect of accumulation of pericardial fluid when either ventricle is failing and so is unable to pull the atrioventricular annulus around the blood column.

Figure 6.3 shows how atrioventricular annular movement augments and supports passive atrial filling in health.

Echocardiography clearly demonstrates exaggerated AVI in action during the early phase of tamponade. The rise in right ventricular pressure during filling causes an exaggerated collapse of the right atrium as it empties. This effect can be seen as a see-sawing motion in Figure 6.4 🔄.

Early signs of haemodynamic compromise

Understanding AVI allows us to explain the early signs of tamponade seen on echo:

Right atrial collapse in diastole: due to exaggerated atrial emptying subsequent to impaired ventricular relaxation.

Right ventricular collapse in diastole: PP exceeds the right ventricular free wall pressure during diastole, causing a geometric change in the ventricular wall, leading to worsening of both diastolic and systolic function.

Initially, the increase in PP causes impairment of relaxation of the right and left ventricles but has little impact on ventricular filling. As the PP continues to rise and exceeds the RAP for part of atrial systole,

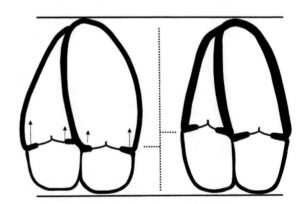

Figure 6.3 **The apex and base are relatively stationary within the thorax during normal respiration.** The longitudinal movement of the annular plane towards the apex in systole creates space for atrial filling, whilst the descent aids ventricular filling.

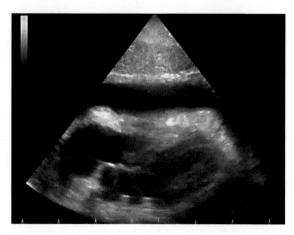

Figure 6.4 [Video 6.1] Subcostal view of a large pericardial effusion demonstrating the exaggerated see-sawing motion of the right ventricular free wall and the right atrium.

This video is available to watch in the online video appendix.

the cardiac output becomes affected and the heart rate will rise in compensation. Symptoms usually start to occur once the PP exceeds 10 mmHg, and almost all patients will be dyspnoeic and tachycardic at 15 mmHg.

Ventricular interdependence and the respiratory cycle

In health, up to a third of the work done by the RV depends upon the LV. To a lesser degree, the LV also relies on a normal RV to function. This phenomenon is due to both the embryological development of muscle fibre orientation in the ventricles, but also the ordered 'sharing' of the interventricular septum during the cardiac cycle.

In health, there is a degree of additional right ventricular filling during inspiration, as the fall in intrapleural pressure with active inspiration sucks blood into the thoracic cavity, filling the right heart. This additional volume is accommodated easily by the healthy intraventricular septum which momentarily moulds to accommodate the extra volume. This effect can be seen echocardiographically as an SV variation of 30% with calm respiration. This effect is illustrated in Figure 6.5.

Progression towards tamponade

The rise in PP seen during cardiac tamponade exaggerates the effect of VI on the interventricular septum. Inspiration fills the RV, and since the free wall cannot

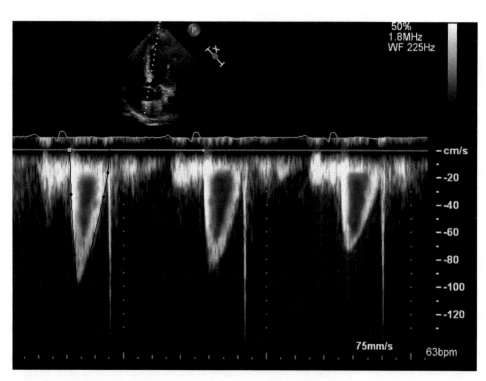

Figure 6.5 Approximately 30% VTI (and SV) variation during normal respiration.

expand due to the accumulated high-pressure pericardial fluid, the septum bows significantly into the LV, distorting the muscle and reducing the ventricular ejection power and potentially reducing filling of the ventricle.

The net effect of this process is to exaggerate the normal SV variation seen with the respiratory cycle, causing the SV to fall with inspiration by a significant proportion.

Blood pressure and left ventricular ejection velocity both fluctuate accordingly, producing the inaptly named clinical sign of **pulsus paradoxus** and transaortic flow variation shown in Figure 6.6.

It is important to note that the same increase in SV variation occurs where there is an abnormally great negative interpleural pressure during inspiration. Where there is high work of breathing due to reduced pulmonary compliance or resistance, the highly negative pressure needed to inspire results in greater SV variation.

The process of tamponade

Tamponade is a medical emergency and can be viewed as the end result of progressive obstructive shock due to cardiac compression. Clinically, it is important to remember that an almost identical physiology may also occur in other clinical situations where there is an acute rise in intrathoracic pressure such as a massive pleural effusion or tension pneumothorax.

When can we say that tamponade has occurred?

The rise in heart rate that accompanies a small effusion does not imply a tamponade but nevertheless signifies compensation for the cardiovascular effect of the effusion.

Figure 6.7 illustrates the rapid fall in SV which occurs at the point at which the PP equalizes with the right ventricular end-diastolic pressure (RVEDP) effectively, dramatically reducing right ventricular filling. From that point, tachycardia is required to maintain an adequate cardiac output, but this alone will not compensate for a progressive rise in PP.

As decompensation progresses and PP approaches 20–25mmHg, the gradient from the mean systemic filling pressure to the right atrium becomes negligible and the atria cannot passively fill. A further rise in PP causes equalization with the left ventricular filling pressure, at which point the SV will fall precipitously and obstructive shock develops. In established tamponade, the diastolic pressures in all chambers are equal and blood cannot flow through the heart.

Figure 6.8 ◖ shows a heart which appears to 'hang' inside the pericardium, stretched by a large effusion, so that the only remaining effect of cardiac motion is to make the heart 'swing' from side to side, producing the sign of 'electrical alternans' seen as a swinging axis on continuous ECG monitoring.

The rate of accumulation dictates how quickly this process advances. Hyperacute 'surgical' effusions

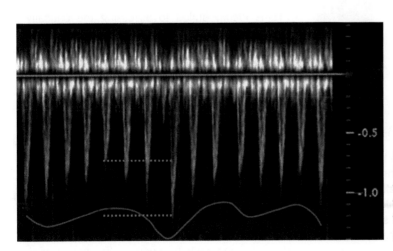

Figure 6.6 Exaggerated left ventricular outflow tract flow variation in tamponade, corresponding to the clinical finding of pulsus paradoxus.

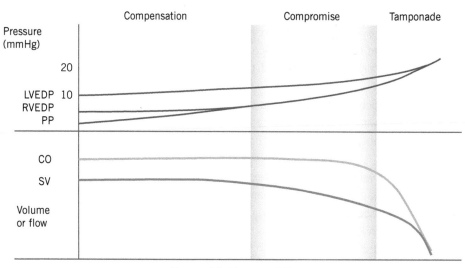

Figure 6.7 Time course of intracardiac and pericardial pressure changes and haemodynamic consequences. CO, cardiac output; LVEDP, left ventricular end-diastolic pressure; PP, pericardial pressure; RVEDP, right ventricular end-diastolic pressure; SV, stroke volume.

arising within minutes can cause a tamponade with as little as 100 mL of fluid, whereas chronic effusions may develop over months and contain >1 L. This differentiation cannot be used as a basis for diagnosis since a chronic non-haemorrhagic effusion may enter a more effusive phase and outstrip the ability of the pericardium to stretch and accommodate it.

It is important to note that the phase of compensation is shorter in patients with hypovolaemia or with a failing RV or an impaired LV. These will be more sensitive to a raised PP and decompensate earlier.

Clinical echocardiographic examination of pericardial fluid

TTE is ideally suited to assessing the critically ill patient with cardiovascular compromise. 2D imaging of the heart will show a section of the pericardium in every standard view, allowing the clinician to rapidly judge the potential impact of an effusion on the clinical context. Be wary of commenting directly on the pericardial thickness, as there is little correlation between the echocardiographic appearance of a thick pericardium and operative or post-mortem findings.

Differentiating fluid from fat and an extra-pericardial haematoma is important. Fat is commonly deposited anterior to the heart, deep to the sternum, and may be seen in the parasternal or

Figure 6.8 [Video 6.2] This figure shows a heart which appears to 'hang' inside the pericardium, stretched by a large effusion, so that the only remaining effect of cardiac motion is to make the heart 'swing' from side to side, producing the sign of 'electrical alternans' seen as a swinging axis on continuous ECG monitoring.

This video is available to watch in the online video appendix.

subcostal views. Occasional accumulation occurs in the atrioventricular and interventricular grooves. It is usually slightly speckled in appearance and will not be seen posteriorly. Fat alone will not affect normal movement of the pericardium. A retrosternal haematoma from surgery or trauma remains anterior to the heart but rarely may compress the RVOT. In trauma, the RV may show regional impairment, in addition.

Examining effusions

Significance of effusion size

Circumferential pericardial effusions are traditionally graded as small, moderate, large, or very large by simple measurement of the deepest region of fluid at end-diastole when the effusion appears at its smallest (Table 6.2). These are descriptive terms and do not imply degrees of haemodynamic significance. The pericardial space should be checked in as many views as possible to assess the extent and distribution of the fluid. Measurements at several points should be documented, acknowledging that a change in patient position may alter the fluid distribution and therefore the repeatability of these findings.

A small effusion will usually be most apparent against the basal infero-lateral border of the LV in the semi-recumbent patient. As more fluid accumulates,

it spreads towards the apex before the anterior and lateral walls are covered. Larger effusions then divide the LA from the descending thoracic aorta, allowing the easy differentiation of pericardial from pleural fluid, as shown in Figures 6.9 and 6.10.

Localized effusions occur in the cardiac surgical setting either early in the form of a haematoma or later due to infection. Rarely, high pulmonary venous pressures can cause an effusion contained within the oblique fissure, potentially resulting in left atrial compression.

In practice, differentiating a pericardial effusion from a large left-sided pleural effusion is important. The key diagnostic feature is based on the anatomical reflection of the pericardium—the oblique sinus—which inserts into the atrio-aortic groove, whereas the pleural reflection is beyond this groove over the surface of the aorta itself.

The diagnostic principle to remember is that in the PLAX view:

* A pleural effusion never separates the aorta from the LA.

In circumstances where a pleural and pericardial effusion coexist, it may be possible to discern the pericardium as a thin white line. This may only be true for the portion perpendicular to the beam.

It is unusual to have an effusion of >500 mL without shortness of breath. An anterior–posterior distance (APD) on PLAX of >12 cm has also been shown to correlate well with the onset of symptoms in chronic

Table 6.2 Categories of effusion size

Size	Depth (mm)	Volume (mL)
Small	<10	<200
Moderate	10–20	200–500 mL
Large	>20	>500 mL
Very large	>20 with chamber compression	500–2000 mL

Data from The Task Force for the Diagnosis and Management of Pericardial Diseases of the European Society of Cardiology (ESC): Adler Y et al., '2015 ESC Guidelines for the diagnosis and management of pericardial diseases', European Heart Journal, 2015, 36, 42, pp. 2921–2964.

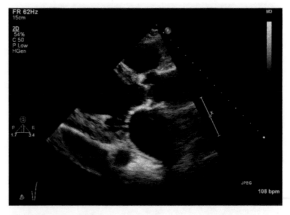

Figure 6.9 Pleural effusions track posteriorly to the descending aorta.

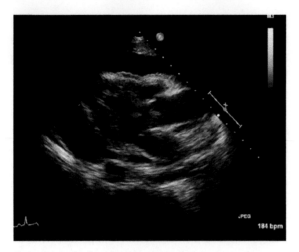

Figure 6.10 Pericardial effusions track between the descending aorta and the left atrium.

effusions. If necessary, the volume present can be estimated using the formula:

$$\text{Volume} = (0.8 \times \text{APD} - 0.6)^3$$

Figure 6.11 illustrates how the APD can be measured.

Practice point

- The absolute size of an effusion may not be significant.
- Make a careful search for signs of an impending tamponade.

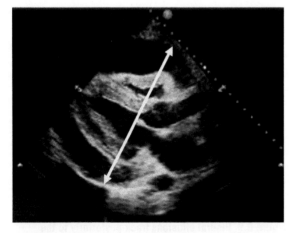

Figure 6.11 The anterior–posterior distance (APD) can be used to estimate the effusion volume.

Echo appearance of pericardial fluid

This is not an exact science, but as a general principle, simple serous or haemorrhagic effusions are generally initially not echogenic and are seen as black spaces. An organized clot may generate 'echo contrast', giving clues to both the cause and treatment. Purulent fluid is usually black, but, as with any effusion relating to longer-term inflammation, echo-dense fibrin stranding may be seen within the effusion.

Discrete masses are rare and are usually artefacts or insignificant cysts but may be a mature haematoma, a tumour, or an infection (particularly fungal).

Practice point

- The appearance of pericardial fluid is not diagnostic alone.

Assessing the haemodynamic significance of pericardial fluid

As with all diagnostic tests, the predictive power of echocardiography depends on the pre-test probability. Table 6.3 lists the most common presenting symptoms of cardiac tamponade in a non-ventilated patient.

In critical care, patients often present with shock, shortness of breath, or a metabolic acidosis, reducing the specificity of these clinical signs for the diagnosis of tamponade. In addition, all the signs of compromise are affected by intrathoracic pressure and also myocardial compliance. For example, significant right

Table 6.3 Clinical features of tamponade in the awake, spontaneously breathing patient

Sign	Sensitivity (approximate %)
Dyspnoea	85–90
Tachycardia	70–85
Pulsus paradoxus	70–90
Elevated jugular venous pressure	65–90
Cardiomegaly on chest radiograph	75–100

ventricular hypertrophy implies a greater PP will be required before ventricular collapse is apparent.

Where a pericardial effusion coexists with critical illness, each echocardiographic sign needs to be judged against our knowledge of the physiology underlying the progression to tamponade.

2D and M-mode

When a pericardial effusion becomes haemodynamically significant, the appearance of an effusion enclosing a hyperdynamic organ with small-chamber dimensions is the most common initial finding. Without overt evidence of haemodynamic compromise, look for the following **sequential** echocardiographic findings as the PP rises.

1. The RA, the chamber with the lowest diastolic pressure, is affected first. Free wall collapse for more than a third of diastole has good sensitivity for tamponade but is non-specific if the collapse does not extend beyond mid-diastole. This appears as a transient concavity of the right atrial wall. M-mode examination of the RA from the subcostal view is often useful to assess this, especially when trying to quantify the duration during tachycardia.

It is common to see spontaneous echo contrast (or 'smoke') within the RA once the cardiac output is compromised. In advanced haemodynamic disturbance, contrast in the form of intravenous agitated saline or colloid can be seen to flow slowly, or even stall, within the RA during spontaneous expiration.

2. The RV is next affected, with diastolic collapse almost always signifying cardiac compromise. The RVOT is usually first affected and may be subtle. Collapse of the free wall follows and is both more obvious and more specific a sign of tamponade.

Again, spontaneous contrast may be seen in the RV, implying reduced cardiac output.

Practice point

The pre-existence of right ventricular hypertrophy can delay these clinical findings, since right ventricular diastolic function is poor at baseline and reset to rely on higher filling pressures. The presence of right ventricular hypertrophy can

also mean that the first impact of tamponade can actually be seen in the left heart.

These echocardiographic findings in the setting of haemodynamic compromise should initiate attempts to drain the pericardial fluid percutaneously or surgically, depending upon the size of the effusion and the clinical context. These findings are more haemodynamically significant if the patient is positive pressure-ventilated.

3. The interventricular septum is affected by the inspiratory swell of the RV. This is not simply an exaggeration of the normal subtle septal movement during respiration but results from an abnormal difference in the filling rates between the ventricles. In effusions causing minimal cardiac impact, there may only be a slight septal 'bounce'. The shift towards the LV becomes more marked as the patient deteriorates and becomes a striking feature which is most clearly visible in the PSAX and four-chamber views.

4. The LA and LV are the last chambers to show diastolic collapse in non-localized effusions, although profound circulatory impairment has often occurred before this is evident on echocardiography.

Small localized effusions most commonly located at the posterior aspect of the LA can cause rapid and catastrophic circulatory collapse. This is seen most often following cardiac surgery and would be an uncommon finding in a general critical care setting. When suspected, TOE or urgent CT is the investigation of choice.

5. The appearance of a 'swinging heart' is the visual representation of the ECG finding of pulsus alternans. Within a large effusion, the heart literally swings with each beat, the pedicle of the pendular motion being the base of the heart, the point of reflection of the serous pericardium.

Doppler studies

Pulsed-wave and continuous-wave Doppler provide valuable information on the direction and velocity of blood flow in all the cardiac chambers and on the impact of respiration.

Intracardiac flow

Exaggerated ventricular interdependence during progression to tamponade gives another tool by which to gauge haemodynamic compromise. Flow variation with respiration is damped on the left side of the heart by the pulmonary vascular bed which acts as a capacity buffer. Without tamponade, flow variation in a normally hydrated person breathing calmly should be:

- <30% variation on the right side of the heart
- <20% variation on the left side of the heart.

Any valve that can be well lined up with a Doppler beam can be used to assess flow variation.

Findings suggestive of circulatory compromise due to an effusion are:

- Increased flow rate during inspiration of >40% across **right**-sided valves or outflow tract
- Decreased flow rate by >25% across **left** heart valves or outflow tract
- Evidence of a restrictive filling pattern in the left heart.

Figures 6.12 and 6.13 show how Doppler should be used to assess respiratory flow variation across a valve; the mitral valve is shown as an example.

Hepatic vein flow

The pattern of blood flow within the hepatic vein is a sensitive and specific method of monitoring the effects of a pericardial effusion.

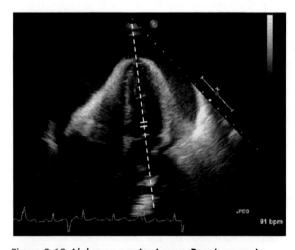

Figure 6.12 Lining up a pulsed-wave Doppler sample area to assess trans-mitral flow variation.

Pulsed-wave Doppler can be used to assess flow direction in diastole and systole in the subcostal view. The hepatic vein joins the IVC just proximal to the junction with the right atrium. If subcostal views are poor or it is too difficult to keep the sample zone inside the vein, then the IVC itself can be used to demonstrate the venous flow pattern in the right ventricular inflow view.

Figure 6.14 demonstrates where Doppler should be placed for assessment of venous patterns in both these positions. And Figure 6.15 shows a normal venous flow pattern.

In a structurally normal heart with neutral fluid balance, flow remains forward in both systole and diastole, giving the 'S' and 'D' waves with a short period of flow reversal during atrial systole's 'a' wave. The flow is often briefly retrograde in between the 'S' and 'D' waves, due to atrial overfilling which generates a small V wave.

In the tamponading heart, abolition of right ventricular passive diastolic filling augments the dependence of the right heart on atrial contraction.

This results in three features of hepatic venous flow in tamponade (Figure 6.16):

1. Pronounced S wave during **inspiration** that reduces in amplitude during **expiration**
2. Diminished 'D' wave during **inspiration** which can disappear altogether, giving an 'adiastolic' flow pattern
3. Large **positive** 'a' waves during expiration.

These effects are the venous reflection of exaggerated respiratory flow variation due to ventricular interdependence. In essence, the bigger the area of wave above the zero flow line, the more significant is the constriction.

Diastolic impairment

In addition to flow variation, Doppler may be used to expose the diastolic dysfunction caused by a haemodynamically significant effusion. Although the time course of diastolic dysfunction in tamponade is as yet unclear, the majority of patients will display a Doppler pattern of moderate or severe diastolic impairment. Pseudonormalization of the MV inflow E and A waves and a tissue Doppler pattern showing diminished E'

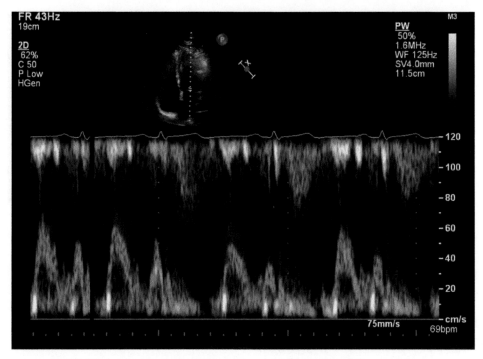

Figure 6.13 Flow variation within a pseudonormal mitral inflow in significant pericardial effusion.

wave (giving a high E/E′ value) are to be expected. In the rare case of effusive constrictive pericarditis where a patient with constrictive pericarditis develops an effusion, both diastology and flow variation become devalued parameters. These patients need specialist review.

Practice point

The reliability of venous flow patterns as a sign of an impending tamponade is abolished by pre-existing high RVEDP in right ventricular hypertrophy and by mechanical ventilation.

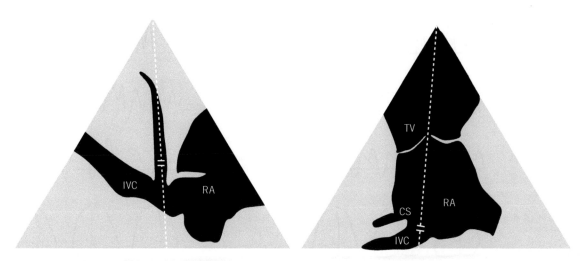

Figure 6.14 Positioning of the pulsed-wave Doppler sample zone to assess hepatic vein flow and IVC flow. IVC, inferior vena cava; RA, right atrium; TV, tricuspid valve; CS, coronary sinus.

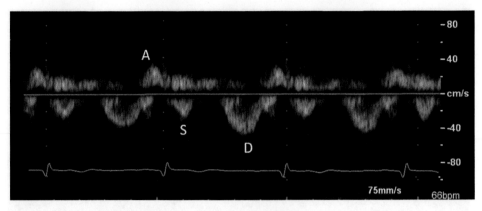

Figure 6.15 Normal hepatic vein or IVC pulsed-wave Doppler flow pattern.

Intracardiac and relevant extracardiac flow wave patterns are summarized in Figure 6.16.

Collating and making sense of findings

All echocardiographic features have varying utility and power for diagnosing and grading the severity of pericardial fluid. Whilst pre-existing structural heart disease and concurrent physiological upset will have an impact on interpretation, the power of the various findings to assess haemodynamic significance are shown in Figure 6.17.

Mechanical ventilation

In the spontaneously ventilating patient, respiration is driven by a fall in intrathoracic pressure. In mechanical ventilation, the reverse is true.

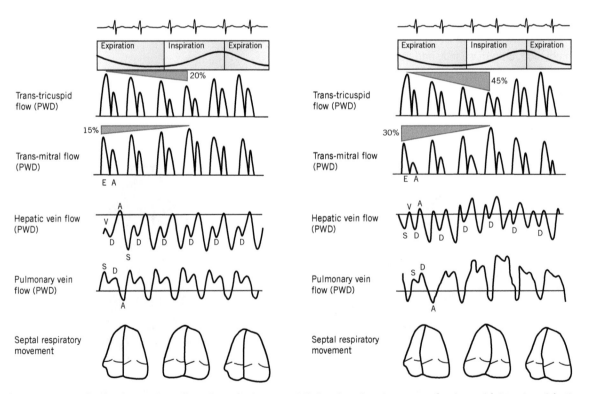

Figure 6.16 Respiration-induced cardiac effects in the normal (left column) and tamponading heart (right column) in the absence of mechanical ventilation. PWD, pulsed-wave Doppler.

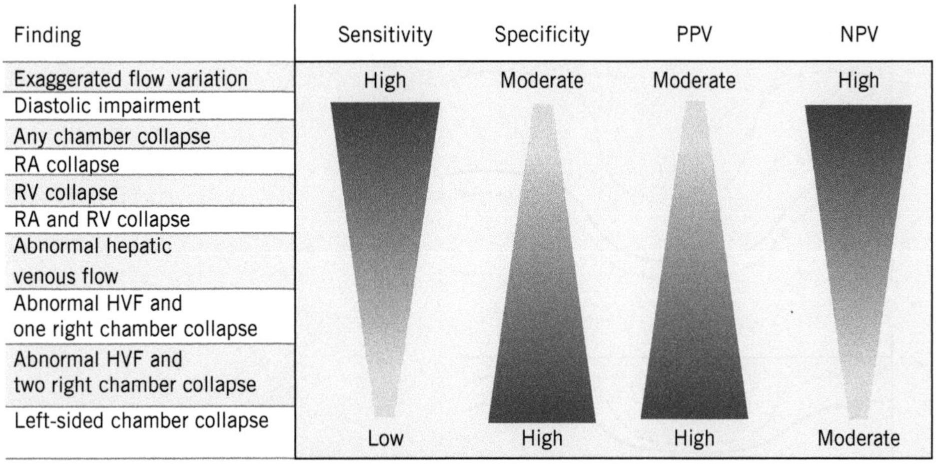

Figure 6.17 Predictive power of chamber collapse and hepatic vein flow pattern in the spontaneously breathing patient. HVF, hepatic vein flow; NPV, negative predictive value; PPV, positive predictive value; RA, right atrium; RV, right ventricle.

Data from Mercé J *et al.*, 'Correlation between clinical and Doppler echocardiographic findings in patients with moderate and large pericardial effusion: implications for the diagnosis of cardiac tamponade', *American Heart Journal*, 1999 Oct;138(4 Pt 1):759–64.

Positive pressure ventilation has significant effects on intrathoracic pressure and therefore on intracardiac pressures. NIV or continuous positive airways pressure (CPAP) delivered at a low level also have a measurable effect on cardiac function. These changes in intrathoracic pressure have a direct effect on cardiac function by altering the pressure relationships between each chamber. The net effect of this cyclical rise in intrathoracic pressure is to:

- Splint the right heart, impairing diastolic function
- Abolish 10–20% of normal right heart filling driven by inspiration
- Drive the septum towards the left ventricular free wall and reduce septal and left ventricular function
- Increase right heart afterload and reduce left ventricular cardiac afterload.

The circulatory consequences of positive pressure ventilation in the presence of a significant pericardial effusion may be seen in Figure 6.18.

The net cardiorespiratory effect of instituting mechanical ventilation is therefore to compound the pressure changes of tamponade. In a patient with pericardial fluid accumulation, institution of mechanical ventilation may therefore **precipitate** tamponade.

Patients who are mechanically ventilated who then develop a significant pericardial effusion represent a significant echocardiographic challenge.

2D imaging signs of tamponade in positive pressure ventilation

These signs are generally thought to hold true with the caveat that as right ventricular diastolic pressure is raised by mechanical ventilation, free wall collapse may be seen at a later stage along the haemodynamic pathway towards tamponade. Consequently, whilst findings may retain specificity, their sensitivity is likely to be reduced.

Flow variation as a sign of tamponade in the positive pressure ventilated patient cannot be relied upon

The impact of positive pressure mechanical ventilation is to raise the RAP and so reduce the filling gradient between the mean systemic filling pressure and the right atrium. This, together with a reduction in negative transmural pressure across the right ventricular free wall, abolishes the augmented filling of the right heart seen with inspiration in the non-ventilated subject. In effect, there is a degree of uncoupling of ventricular interdependence, making flow variation

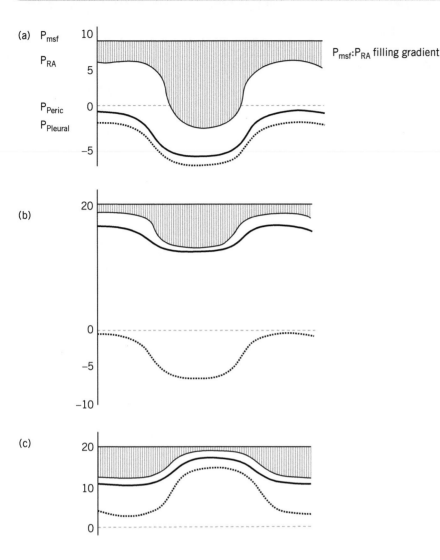

Figure 6.18 **Right atrial pressure and filling and its relation to pericardial and pleural pressures (a) in health, (b) in tamponade during spontaneous breathing, and (c) in tamponade during mechanical ventilation.** P_{msf}, mean systemic filling pressure; P_{RA}, right atrial pressure; P_{Peric}, pericardial pressure; $P_{Pleural}$, pleural pressure.

in positive pressure ventilation more dependent on filling and the afterload seen independently by each ventricle.

Clinically, therefore, it is vital to add this to our diagnostic thought processes.

Practice point

In the patient on mechanical ventilation, the pragmatic approach is to err on the side of assuming that any circulatory instability in the presence of a significant or rapidly accumulated effusion is due to an impending cardiac tamponade. Flow variation is confounded and should not be used. Expert consensus should be sought where possible.

The following case study illustrates some of these points.

CASE STUDY

The use of echocardiography for assessing the haemodynamic impact of a pericardial effusion in the context of mechanical ventilation

The intensive care team were called to see a 33-year-old woman who had recently received chemotherapy for acute leukaemia. She required rapid intubation for respiratory failure. Her chest X-ray following intubation and ventilation showed bibasal shadowing consistent with atelectasis and pleural fluid, and her blood pressure was 80/50 mmHg, with a heart rate of 120 bpm. Over the

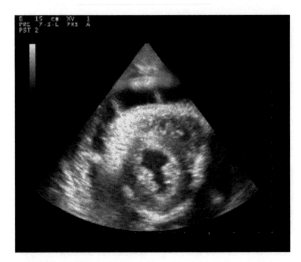

Figure 6.19 Fibrin strands are evident in the complex moderate pericardial effusion.

following 3 hours, the intensive care team attempted to optimize her circulation with fluid boluses and low-dose noradrenaline. Despite initial improvement, her blood pressure deteriorated to 70/35 mmHg. Further information about her cardiovascular state was sought, and a TTE demonstrated a pericardial effusion which was moderate in size, with fibrinous stranding, as shown in Figure 6.19.

There was significant collapse of the right atrium during diastole, but no flow variation across the RVOT or LVOT. Following further fluid boluses and commencement of adrenaline, the patient's blood pressure fell to 75 mmHg systolic and her heart rate peaked at 155 bpm. The team concluded that despite the lack of classical echocardiographic findings, the diagnosis was cardiac tamponade.

The cardiology team were called, agreed with the clinical assessment, and assisted with the placement of a Seldinger pericardial drain from the subcostal position. Following initial drainage of 50 mL of thick, turbid fluid, the intensive care team rapidly weaned the adrenaline infusion, with an improvement in blood pressure and a reduction in heart rate from 155 to 100 bpm. However, the drain was problematic and haemodynamic instability reoccurred within a further 6 hours. A further 50 mL was aspirated with some difficulty, and the patient was taken to theatre for surgical decompression, formation of a pericardial window, and insertion of a large-bore drain.

Decompression

Decision-making

The path to deciding to drain pericardial fluid is altered in acute severe illness. The following factors should be taken into account when making a decision of whether or not, or when, to drain an effusion:

- The presence or likelihood of complication by further cardiovascular stressors, for example the patient with compensatory tachycardia may not be able to maintain cardiac output if they become pyrexial
- Pre-existing comorbidities affecting progression to tamponade:
  - Cardiac, for example pre-existing poor left ventricular function
  - Non-cardiac: calcification of the capacitance vessels due to radiotherapy
- Balance of risk according to the patient's current coagulation status
- Thoracic anatomical abnormality, for example pectus excavatum
- Mental state balanced against the safety of sedation, or even potentially highly risky tracheal intubation, to increase the chance of success
- Likelihood of effective needle drainage vs the need for a pericardial window:
  - Tamponade due to slowly accumulating blood
  - Tamponade due to a pyopericardium.

Surgical pericardiotomy should be carefully considered in the following circumstances:

- Anatomical variation making needle pericardiocentesis impossible
- Haemopericardium due to trauma or localized post-surgical pericardial collections
- Loculated effusions
- Pyopericardium
- Requirement for a biopsy.

The urgency of decompression is dictated by the clinical trend. Drainage in controlled conditions using echocardiographic guidance is preferable when time and facilities allow. Rapid progression to tamponade may make immediate drainage of part, or all, of the fluid lifesaving.

The risks of arrhythmia, vagal surges, pneumothorax, bowel or liver injury, and myocardial laceration or arterial injury must all be acknowledged, although it is very unlikely that formal consent can be obtained prior to emergency fluid drainage. Because of the likelihood of progression in large effusions caused by neoplasia, tuberculous disease, uraemia, hypothyroidism, and parasitic disease, some centres recommend drainage when the depth exceeds 20 mm (in diastole) in an elective setting, whether or not fluid or biopsy is needed for diagnosis.

The following case study illustrates some of these points.

CASE STUDY

The role of echocardiography in the diagnosis and treatment of acute cardiac tamponade

A 64-year-old man with a known chronic pericardial effusion related to rheumatoid arthritis presented with symptomatic complete heart block after minor elective surgery.

An emergency temporary pacing wire was inserted, although it was a difficult procedure.

Despite good pacing capture and a brief improvement in symptoms, the patient became dyspnoeic and agitated and collapsed on the floor of the cardiology ward. The jugular venous pressure was obviously raised, and the intensive care team was fast-paged to the patient in a peri-arrest state with an unrecordable blood pressure and agitation. The pacing wire was now failing to capture, and the heart rate was 45 bpm.

The airway was maintained manually, and spontaneous breathing gently supported with a bag–valve mask. Echo demonstrated a circumferential 2.0-cm pericardial effusion. The right atrium was collapsed almost throughout the cardiac cycle in the apical view and the RV was seen to collapse in diastole, whilst the LA was also filling poorly, as shown in the parasternal view (Figures 6.20 ⬤ and 6.21).

Continuous-wave Doppler placed across the tricuspid valve showed a large variation in velocity with respiration. The pacing wire could be seen within the effusion around the RV, and it was felt that ventricular perforation and bleeding into the pericardium had led to tamponade.

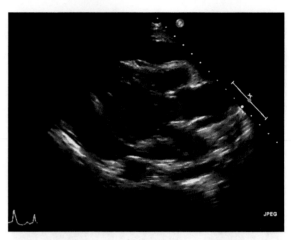

Figure 6.20 [Video 6.3] Right ventricular outflow collapse is evident and the late signs of partial left atrial collapse and an underfilled left ventricle are present.
⬤ *This video is available to watch in the online video appendix.*

Boluses of 100 micrograms of adrenaline were given intravenously, whilst the patient was lifted onto a bed, and external pacing pads were applied and set to a rate of 70 bpm at 70 J. An emergency needle pericardiocentesis kit was opened. A sterile field was set up and the echo probe was covered with a sterile sheath. Sterile aqua-gel was used to obtain a subcostal view. A second member of the team inserted the needle into the pericardial space alongside the echo probe in line with the plane of view. Once the needle was observed to enter the space, 2 mL

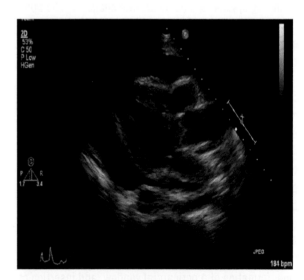

Figure 6.21 The characteristic 'kinked' appearance of right ventricular collapse during diastole in tamponade.

of saline were injected. Bubbles and fluid movement were seen in the pericardial space. A total of 20 mL of blood were removed; the needle was kept in place, whilst the blood pressure was rechecked. Some improvement was noted; a further 20 mL of blood were removed, and the blood pressure improved to 100/60 mmHg. The needle was removed.

The patient was moved to the cardiac catheter lab, and a further echocardiogram performed. Fluid remained in the pericardial space, with evidence of ongoing right ventricular and right atrial collapse. A Seldinger drain was inserted under echo guidance, and a new pacing wire was inserted.

Over the next 6 hours, the drain output tailed off and the drain was removed the following day.

Procedure for emergency pericardiocentesis

The two most common approaches to drainage are the subcostal, followed by the apical (through the rib space below, and 1cm lateral to, the apex). Echo guidance should be used to reveal the most accessible or deepest section of the effusion, as shown in Figure 6.22, and also to estimate the best trajectory, avoiding unnecessary perforation of organs. For example, the view should be unimpaired by expanding lungs **throughout** the respiratory cycle; the tidal volume or inflation pressures can often be reduced temporarily to allow a larger window in the mechanically ventilated patient.

Pressure can be temporarily or permanently relieved using a needle mounted on a syringe and a three-way tap. The needle will not always be sonographically visible. Once the needle is thought to be within the fluid, a small volume of agitated saline or colloid can be given as a form of contrast. The appearance of the contrast within the pericardium confirms correct placement.

Use of the Seldinger technique to insert a drain over a guide-wire should be considered and is a requisite in acute haemopericardium since rapid re-accumulation is likely prior to definitive management.

Initial aspiration of just a few millilitres may give dramatic clinical improvement in the acute setting. If a drain is left *in situ*, it is advisable to titrate the drainage rate to cardiovascular parameters and reduce the rate once circulatory stability is achieved, as rapid large volume removal can lead to paradoxical haemodynamic instability whilst central venous filling pressures restabilize. The drain remains *in situ* for intermittent manual aspiration, which may be necessary every few hours in thicker effusions. It may be removed once the rate has fallen to levels of <25 mL per 24 hours.

Summary algorithm

Figure 6.23 is intended to summarize everything discussed in this chapter and act as an aide-memoire in clinical practice.

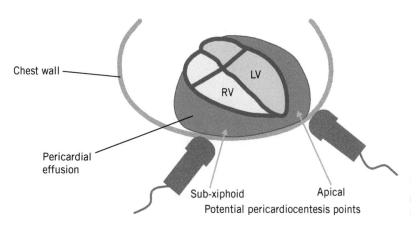

Chest wall

LV

RV

Pericardial effusion

Sub-xiphoid   Apical

Potential pericardiocentesis points

Figure 6.22 Standard access points for pericardial drainage.

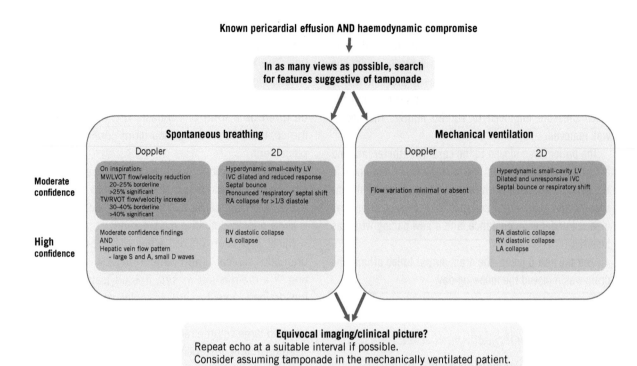

Known pericardial effusion AND haemodynamic compromise

In as many views as possible, search for features suggestive of tamponade

Spontaneous breathing

	Doppler	2D
Moderate confidence	On inspiration: MV/LVOT flow/velocity reduction 20–25% borderline >25% significant TV/RVOT flow/velocity increase 30–40% borderline >40% significant	Hyperdynamic small-cavity LV IVC dilated and reduced response Septal bounce Pronounced 'respiratory' septal shift RA collapse for >1/3 diastole
High confidence	Moderate confidence findings AND Hepatic vein flow pattern - large S and A, small D waves	RV diastolic collapse LA collapse

Mechanical ventilation

	Doppler	2D
Moderate confidence	Flow variation minimal or absent	Hyperdynamic small-cavity LV Dilated and unresponsive IVC Septal bounce or respiratory shift
High confidence		RA diastolic collapse RV diastolic collapse LA collapse

Equivocal imaging/clinical picture?
Repeat echo at a suitable interval if possible.
Consider assuming tamponade in the mechanically ventilated patient.

Figure 6.23 Summary algorithm. The echocardiographic features of circulatory compromise due to a pericardial effusion, and their diagnostic power.

Multiple choice questions

1. Sensitive signs of circulatory compromise due to pericardial effusion include:
   A Posterior pericardial effusion depth of 2 cm
   B Right atrial diastolic collapse during mechanical ventilation
   C Left atrial diastolic collapse
   D Inspiratory collapse of the inferior vena cava
   E Markers of left ventricular diastolic impairment

2. Echocardiographic signs of tamponade with good specificity include:
   A Right atrial collapse
   B Septal dyskinesia
   C Left atrial collapse
   D Trans-mitral velocity variation of >30%
   E Abnormal hepatic vein flow and right ventricular collapse

3. In the presence of a pericardial effusion, flow variation across valves or outflow tracts:

A Does not require the Doppler beam to be well aligned to flow
B Is greater in the right heart than the left heart
C Provides a sensitive measure of circulatory compromise during spontaneous respiration
D Provides a sensitive measure of circulatory compromise during mechanical ventilation
E Is affected by work of breathing

4. The differential diagnosis for the echocardiographic appearance of a pericardial effusion includes:
   A Pleural effusion
   B Extracardiac fat
   C Pericardial tumours
   D Retrosternal haematoma
   E Left ventricular pseudoaneurysm

5. Regarding percutaneous drainage of pericardial effusions:
   A Echocardiography may be used to identify the safest approach
   B Echocardiography alone may be used to justify urgent drainage

C The needle is often not visible on the screen

D A small amount of agitated saline may be used as contrast to confirm the needle is in the pericardial space

E Echocardiography is a substitute for expertise

For answers to multiple choice questions, please see 'Appendix 1: Answers to multiple choice questions', p. 171.

Further reading

Armstrong WF, Ryan T. Cardiac tamponade. In: Armstrong WF, Ryan T. *Feigenbaum's Echocardiography*, 7th edition. Lippincott Williams and Wilkins, Philadelphia, 2010, pp. 248–51.

Bodson L, Bouferrache K, Vieillard-Baron A. Cardiac tamponade. *Curr Opin Crit Care* 2011; **17**: 416–24.

Faehnrich JA, Noone RB, White WD, *et al*. Effects of positive-pressure ventilation, pericardial effusion, and cardiac tamponade on respiratory variation in transmitral flow velocities. *J Cardiothorac Vasc Anesth* 2003; **17**: 45–50.

Maisch B, Seferović PM, Ristić AD, *et al*. Guidelines on the diagnosis and management of pericardial diseases executive summary; The Task force on the diagnosis and management of pericardial diseases of the European Society of Cardiology. *Eur Heart J* 2004; **25**: 587–610.

Sharp JT, Bunnell IL, Holland JF, Griffith GT, Greene DG. Hemodynamics during induced cardiac tamponade in man. *Am J Med* 1960; **29**: 640–6.

Tsang TS, Oh JK, Seward JB. Diagnosis and management of cardiac tamponade in the era of echocardiography. *Clin Cardiol* 1999; **22**: 446–52.

7

Volume assessment and fluid responsiveness

The importance of volume assessment

Contemporary practice in resuscitating the critically ill necessitates accurate and continuing assessment of fluid requirements. Assessment of intravascular volume remains a complex area. Clinical signs of hypovolaemia due to haemorrhage may remain masked for some time in the young, fit patient; yet fluid overload in the post-acute phase of critical illness is associated with organ dysfunction, increased length of stay, and more days on the ventilator.

Critical care echo should always be performed to answer a clinical question. When using echocardiography to assess the intravascular volume status, you need to understand the clinical context to ask the right clinical question. For example, the hypotensive trauma patient and the hypotensive patient with septic shock may both benefit from fluid, but the echocardiographic findings and the context will be quite different.

Haemorrhagic, cardiogenic, distributive, and obstructive shock all demonstrate individual cardiac physiology, and the risks of inadequate and excessive resuscitation are different.

The volume of blood required to fill the vessels and the additional volume required to generate a systemic filling pressure, the unstressed and stressed volumes, vary considerably in health and illness. A patient with haemorrhage is likely to have low volume within both compartments, whereas a septic patient in distributive shock may have a large blood volume in the vasodilated capacitance vessels, but a much lower stressed central volume. Delivering fluid may temporarily improve cardiac output in both, but haemostasis and reversal of vasoplegia, respectively, are the ultimate cure. In cardiogenic and obstructive shock, fluid is usually not a significant part of the solution.

Repeated studies have shown that 'end-of-the-bed' clinical suspicion that volume loading will improve cardiac output is correct only half of the time in the general critically ill population. Crucially, understanding cardiovascular physiology through echocardiography enhances our awareness that blood pressure as a function of vasoconstriction does not equate to, and is often to the detriment of, delivered stroke volume—the heart cannot continue to eject blood adequately when the circulation is super-constricted. Echocardiography is the only tool we have in critical care which fully describes a patient's position on the Frank–Starling curve. Figure 7.1 shows how important this is by showing the different curve shapes for a heart with normal, reduced, and hyperdynamic circulations.

> **Practice point**
> Understanding individual ventricular function is key to assessing fluid responsiveness.

Volume and timing of fluid delivery

Assessing fluid responsiveness is not the same as examining intravascular volume. For example, where the ventricle is failing, the patient may have a low central blood volume and yet be unresponsive to fluid. It is not requisite that critically ill patients should reside at the peak of their Frank–Starling curve. Fluid responsiveness has therefore come to be defined as:

' . . . an increase in cardiac output or stroke volume of 10 to 15% following delivery of 500 millilitres of fluid over 15 minutes.'

The critical care literature describes two phases to fluid administration. In the early resuscitation phase,

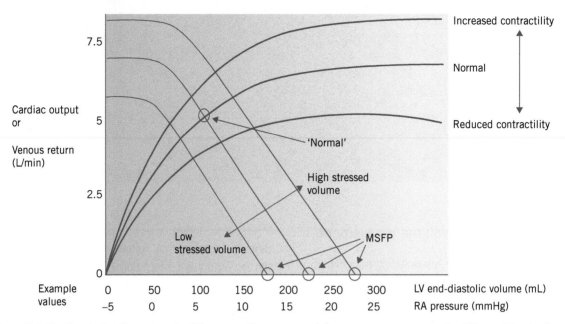

Figure 7.1 The Frank–Starling curves in different cardiac states and the venous return curves for different blood volume distributions. LV, left ventricle; RV, right ventricle; MSFP, mean systemic filling pressure.

measured in hours, there is a clear message that fluid under-resuscitated is detrimental to patient survival.

There is, however, mounting evidence that a more conservative approach to fluid administration is appropriate beyond the early resuscitation period. This has been predominantly studied in conditions such as acute lung injury and AKI and in the perioperative period for bowel surgery. Adverse effects of inadequate volume are usually evident early, whereas the effects of excessive volume are often more insidious but similarly deleterious.

Beyond the resuscitation period, the patient with acute septic shock or pancreatitis needs more frequent assessment of fluid requirements than, for example, a patient with an exacerbation of chronic obstructive pulmonary disease in the process of being weaned from mechanical ventilation. Nevertheless, the principles remain the same.

When deciding to give fluid, any potential improvement in cardiac output should be weighed against the harm of giving additional fluid. The pulmonary capillary endothelium becomes more permeable to water during the inflammatory response; extravascular lung water therefore rises, in relation to the delivered volume, more acutely than in health, as shown in Figure 7.2.

Endothelial injury is not restricted to pulmonary capillaries. The inflammatory response damages the vital glycocalyx layer on the capillary endothelium normally preserving cell-to-cell contact and controlling fluid permeability. Fluid boluses with a crystalloid further strip the glycocalyx, leading to widespread endothelial dysfunction and the tendency to form oedema. As well as pulmonary congestion, which has a direct impact upon the length of ventilatory support, renal, neurological, and gastrointestinal functions are also impaired by over-resuscitation with fluid.

> **Practice point**
>
> The importance of fluid responsiveness varies according to the phase of critical illness and must be interpreted within the clinical context.

Static and dynamic markers of fluid responsiveness

A static marker of fluid response is a measurement taken without disturbing the system at one point in time. Historically, prediction of response to fluid has relied on static haemodynamic markers such as central venous pressure, RAP, pulmonary artery occlusion pressure, and measurement of left or right ventricular end-diastolic

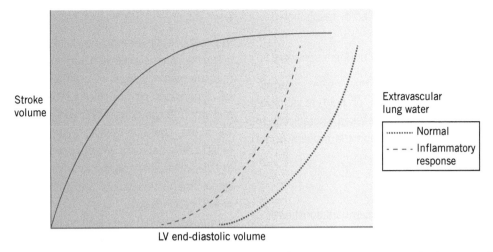

Figure 7.2 The effect of rising end-diastolic volume and, by assumption, pressure on extravascular lung water in the normal lung and during systemic inflammation.

dimensions using echocardiography. In practice, these measurements have been used in sequential assessment of response to fluid aliquots, estimating the position of the left ventricular myocardial stretch on the Frank–Starling curve. Overall, the literature on fluid responsiveness has shown that simply knowing the preload status does not improve our ability to predict a response to fluid.

Features suggestive of high left ventricular atrial pressures are other static markers that may support a projected lack of benefit from fluid loading. If pulsed-wave Doppler examination of the mitral inflow pattern and pulmonary vein flow and tissue Doppler of the mitral annulus suggest a significantly elevated left ventricular filling pressure, then beneficial response to fluid is unlikely. This use of such parameters is not yet substantially validated and is the subject of ongoing research.

Additionally, it is suspected that the presence of elevated LVOT velocities sometimes represents impaired flow that may be improved by fluid loading. Patients with asymmetric ventricular hypertrophy or other regional hypertrophy are known to be at risk of dynamic outflow tract obstruction, including encroachment of the aMVL into the LVOT, but it is reasonable to assume that those with lesser degrees of asymmetry are also at risk in low-volume or hyperdynamic states. This group may include borderline hypertrophy, proximal septal hypertrophy (common in the elderly), or even an apparently normal ventricle that behaves abnormally under hypovolaemic or distributive shock conditions. The reason

for identifying these patients is that improving the circulating volume may have a disproportionate benefit through improved outflow tract dynamics.

In general, however, when using echocardiography, simple LV dimensions or end-diastolic volume estimation are likely to remain reasonable markers of low circulating volume when they are at or below their lower limits, **and** pathology leading to obstructive shock is not present. Nevertheless, overall clinical practice has moved away from static markers towards the practice of forecasting fluid responsiveness using a dynamic aspect of the circulation. Dynamic markers of fluid responsiveness are measurements taken during 'provocation' of the circulation. This is commonly achieved either using the interaction of the respiratory cycle or a change in posture to provide a surrogate fluid challenge. These markers can be evaluated using TTE.

Practice point

Markers of preload are not markers of preload responsiveness.

The physiology underlying echo assessment of fluid responsiveness

Echocardiography provides a non-invasive method of haemodynamic assessment using:

1. Absolute measurements of chamber dimensions

2. Changes in blood flow provoked by respiration or posture change

3. Large vein diameter variation during respiration.

Although echocardiography may give intermittent information, the question of fluid responsiveness is usually posed and addressed sporadically to determine a direction of care and the process is not time-consuming.

Chamber dimensions

Given that the size of cardiac chambers constitutes a static marker of filling, it is not surprising that simple assessment of dimensions is generally both insensitive and poorly specific.

However, in significant hypovolaemia, the end-systolic diameter of the LV will be diminished relative to its pre-morbid size. In an otherwise normal LV, continued blood volume decrease causes the papillary muscles to oppose or 'kiss', eventually obliterating the cavity as the heart rate accelerates, eventually leading to cardiovascular collapse and arrest.

The left ventricular end-diastolic dimension might also be expected to be small in hypovolaemia, but this requires knowledge of the patient's left ventricular size in health. Change in the left ventricular end-diastolic area in response to filling is closer to a dynamic marker and is commonly used in intra-operative echo to guide fluid administration during periods of blood loss or significant fluid shifts. This method, however, lacks specificity, given that the end-diastolic area is also a component of myocardial stretch and capacitance, and therefore a reflection of the underlying diastolic function. Indeed, the presence of diastolic dysfunction necessitates caution when fluid loading, as a higher rise in pulmonary venous pressure would be expected relative to a normal LV.

Looking at the right atrial and ventricular size may add supportive information in the setting of gross hypovolaemia, but the causes of a dilated right heart are diverse and usually pressure-, and not volume-, related. Fluid status should therefore not be inferred in isolation from right heart dimensions. In particular, the presence of septal flattening suggests that fluid will be poorly tolerated as left ventricular impingement would be likely to worsen.

Limitations

In general, hypovolaemia needs to be profound before it is evident on simple visual assessment or diameter measurement. Normal or large left or right ventricular dimensions do not rule out profound hypovolaemia where those dimensions had not been previously examined. Low end-systolic volumes, although more reliable as a marker of gross hypovolaemia, also occurs in LVH, obstructive shock such as tamponade or PE, significant vasodilatation, and with high endogenous or induced inotropy.

Intra-abdominal pressure can have an independent effect on the calibre of the IVC which is not related to fluid status. Raised intra-abdominal pressure can cause artificial flattening of the IVC. Exaggerated respiratory effort may also cause a misleading degree of IVC collapse.

Stroke volume variation with respiration

Preload changes during respiration result in cyclical changes in SV, predominantly due to changes in left ventricular end-diastolic volume. This can be used as a tool for dynamic assessment of fluid responsiveness using echocardiography.

Heart–lung interaction and venous return

During spontaneous inspiration, negative intra-pleural pressure induces a gradient between the systemic filling pressure and the right atrium, and blood flows into the right heart. The right atrium is a thin-walled capacitance chamber and it swells in response to the increased filling. This function of the right atrium feeds the RV with volume during ventricular diastole, augmenting the SV. Blood then passes through the pulmonary circulation in between 1 and 4 s, depending upon cardiac output. The LV then receives this rise in venous return from the pulmonary veins. This phenomenon of heart–lung interaction results in a breath-to-breath Stroke Volume Variation (SVV) of around 20–30% in health whilst breathing at rest.

These pressure changes are shown in Figure 7.3.

Effect of mechanical ventilation on heart–lung interaction and venous return

During full mechanical ventilation without any intrinsic respiratory effort, the normal heart–lung interaction

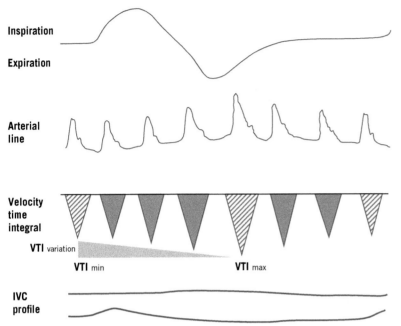

Figure 7.3 **Circulatory parameter variation during spontaneous variation.** VTI, velocity time integral; IVC, inferior vena cava.

and effect on venous return are both **inverted and blunted**.

Lung expansion is now driven by positive intrathoracic pressure which causes compression of the heart and great vessels to a degree related to inflation pressures and the tidal volume. The lower native right heart pressures are therefore affected to a greater degree through:

1. Reduction in venous return: preload
2. Pulmonary vascular bed compression: afterload
3. Direct compression of the RV.

The net effect of this is reduced right ventricular filling, and then in turn, reduced left ventricular stroke volume. This inverted variation in SV with respiration is usually 15–20% during mechanical ventilation in a euvolaemic patient without cardiac compromise.

We can use this physiology to assess fluid responsiveness. A low SVV of 10% suggests that cardiac function is approaching the apex of the Starling curve. A value of 10-15% should be viewed as a grey zone, meaning that other supportive evidence should be sought. An SVV of >15% suggests great fluid responsiveness and therefore that cardiac stretch currently resides on the steeper part of the Starling curve. This is shown in Figure 7.4.

SVV has been shown to be an accurate and repeatable reflection of fluid responsiveness. Studies have shown both sensitivity and specificity of SVV in the mechanically ventilated patient to be in excess of 80%, with an area under the receiver–operator curve of at least 0.9.

> **Practice point**
>
> An SVV of 15% or above is strongly suggestive of fluid responsiveness. An SVV of <10% suggests that fluid responsiveness is unlikely.

This flow and blood velocity variation can be assessed using a number of techniques, including Doppler echocardiography, specifically employing pulsed-wave Doppler.

Limitations

In practice, a potential source of error is movement of the heart due to respiration. For example, using the apical five-chamber view, the sample point for pulsed-wave Doppler may move basally and apically within the LVOT by as much as a centimetre during the respiratory cycle. This effect can artefactually increase flow variation. This may be attenuated by temporarily

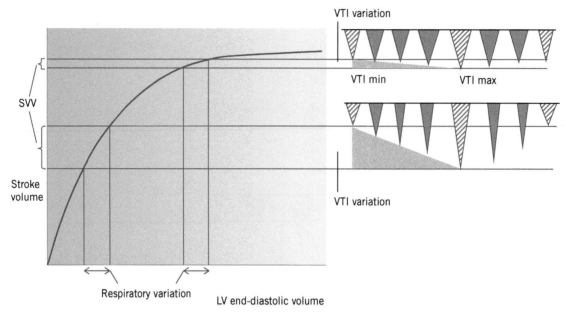

Figure 7.4 The difference in stroke volume variation, depending on which part of the Frank–Starling curve the patient resides. SVV, stroke volume variation.

altering ventilation settings or it may prompt the use of another assessment method.

Arrhythmias inherently lead to large stroke volume variation. Much longer sample times can be applied, but this becomes logistically difficult, time-consuming, and inaccurate where the difference between fluid responsiveness and non-fluid responsiveness is as little as 5%. SVV should not therefore be used in the setting of arrhythmias.

Tidal volume also affects flow and velocity variation. Tidal volumes of <6 ml/kg or >8 ml/kg induce smaller or larger degrees of variation in SV, potentially reducing the predictive power of SVV as a marker of fluid responsiveness. Brief alteration of tidal volumes into the range of 6 to 8 ml/kg to optimize the value of assessment may be acceptable.

The use of negatively chronotropic agents has also been shown to affect the validity of SVV by artificially increasing the diastolic filling time and augmenting the SV.

Posture-induced capacitance volume changes

Raising the legs from the horizontal position to 45 degrees causes transient movement of lower limb venous blood towards the heart, mimicking a fluid bolus. This provides a 'stressed volume' load of between 150 and 300 mL to the central circulation. The increase in cardiac output due to increased myocardial stretch peaks at about 90 s and is gone within a few minutes.

The manoeuvre can be achieved in one of two ways, depending on the initial position of the patient, as shown in Figure 7.5. Measurement of the increment in cardiac output or equivalent is done before and after passive leg raising. A number of studies and reviews have demonstrated the maintenance of reliability of this manoeuvre, even in the setting of arrhythmias and spontaneous respiratory effort on a ventilator, making it a useful tool in these two groups of people.

> **Practice point**
>
> A 5–10% rise in cardiac output or SV is a reasonable indicator of fluid responsiveness for clinical use. More than 10% increase in cardiac output strongly suggests fluid responsiveness. Less than 5% change in cardiac output makes fluid responsiveness very unlikely.

Limitations

Passive leg raising is occasionally not possible due to restrictions on patient positioning. In other groups

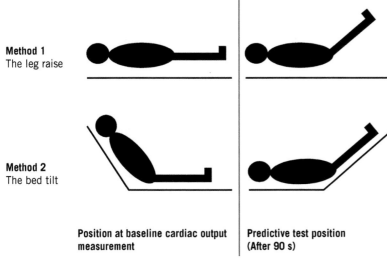

Method 1
The leg raise

Method 2
The bed tilt

| Position at baseline cardiac output measurement | Predictive test position (After 90 s) |

Figure 7.5 **The two predominant methods for performing a passive leg raise.**

of patients, the act of repositioning has potential to induce either pain, and consequently a sympathetic response, or respiratory compromise—each of which may affect the validity of the test.

High-dose vasopressor use, severe peripheral vascular disease, raised intra-abdominal pressure, and more obviously previous lower limb amputation are thought to reduce the sensitivity of this test.

A further issue is the effect on obtaining echocardiographic images once the new position is adopted. If an alternative view, for example the RVOT as opposed to the LVOT, is required, then repeatability error may be introduced.

Central vein diameter variability

In health, normal inspiration results in a degree of collapse of the abdominal inferior cava and a degree of distension of the thoracic superior vena cava. During positive pressure ventilation without spontaneous effort, these changes are reversed. Increased RAP during positive pressure inspiration reduces the gradient between mean upstream pressure and the central veins. The extent of this compression or distension depends upon the amount and distribution of the intrathoracic pressure, as well as the intra-abdominal pressure.

The respiratory variation of the size of the central veins cannot be reliably used for fluid responsiveness assessment in the presence of spontaneous respiratory effort. In the patient not undergoing any form of

positive pressure ventilation, the size and collapsibility of the inferior cava reflects only the RAP, which is unhelpful for gauging fluid responsiveness. However, a very small collapsing vessel does suggest that a fluid load will at least be tolerated.

In patients with assisted ventilation who are at least triggering each breath, the interpretation of IVC size variability is difficult. Although once again, it is probable that the small and collapsing vessel continues to suggest hypovolaemia and fluid tolerance, and the large unvarying vessel predicts no benefit from volume loading and potential harm.

In the fully ventilated patient with no respiratory effort, the degree of IVC diameter variation through the respiratory cycle is useful in the prediction of fluid responsiveness. The less the variation, the less likely the patient is to respond favourably to fluid loading.

> **Practice point**
>
> Interpreting the IVC according to the mechanism of ventilation:
> - Respiratory variation of the size of the central veins cannot be reliably used for fluid responsiveness assessment in the presence of spontaneous respiratory effort
> - In a patient not undergoing any form of positive pressure ventilation, the size and collapsibility of the inferior cava reflects the RAP:

- If the IVC diameter is <1.5 cm and varies >50%, the RAP is usually below 5 mmHg
- If the IVC diameter is >2 cm and varies <50%, the RAP is likely to be above 15 mmHg, which is unhelpful for gauging fluid responsiveness
- However, in a spontaneously breathing or triggering patient, a very small collapsing vessel does suggest that a fluid load will be tolerated
- By removing all respiratory effort, full mechanical ventilation creates ideal conditions for interpreting IVC diameter variation as a marker of fluid responsiveness.

Limitations

IVC diameter variability is externally affected by both high intra-abdominal pressure and abnormally high or low interpleural pressure. When ventilation is not fully mechanically controlled, we cannot interpret the behaviour of the IVC as solely reflecting fluid responsiveness in the capacitance vessels. In conditions resulting in high respiratory effort, variability would be expected to be falsely high. When respiratory effort is weak, such as in a tiring patient, it may be that variability is falsely low. Additionally, IVC analysis will not be reliable in right heart hypertrophy or dysfunction, particularly when septal movement is impaired.

Practical approach to assessment of fluid responsiveness in the critically ill

The clinical question being asked should be clear before you select your assessment approach:

1. Is there frank hypovolaemia?
2. Will cardiac output improve with fluid—is there evidence of fluid responsiveness?
3. Will fluid removal be tolerated?

Frank hypovolaemia

Key echocardiographic markers of severe hypovolaemia:

1. A hyperdynamic LV with low end-systolic volume or even papillary apposition may be present.

End-systolic diameter can be checked against the normal range corrected for BSA. End-diastolic volume may also be low, although this is more difficult to recognize. These measurements can be made reliably in the parasternal long axis, parasternal short axis, and subcostal long axis views. Other views may be used when necessary, acknowledging the additional potential inaccuracy

2. In the parasternal short axis view, a cross-sectional area at the mid-left ventricular level of <10 cm² is technically low. The value corrected for BSA is 5.5 cm²/m²

3. A very small IVC diameter is strongly indicative of severe hypovolaemia:

   a. In the non-ventilated patient, look for a diameter of <1.0 cm with collapse on **inspiration**

   b. In the ventilated patient, splinting of venous cardiac inflow by mechanical ventilation means that the same degree of hypovolaemia is present with a vena caval diameter of <1.5 cm with evidence of collapse on **expiration**

4. A patient with an IVC that collapses by 50% or more or who has a low end-diastolic volume can safely be assumed to be fluid-tolerant.

CASE STUDY

The use of bedside echocardiography in resuscitation

An 18-year-old man was brought into the emergency department after falling from scaffolding. He had no significant past medical history. On arrival, his airway and cervical spine raised no concerns. His respiratory rate was 24 breaths per minute and he complained of considerable pain in his right lumbar region. His heart rate was 118 bpm and blood pressure on arrival was 105/55 mmHg. His peripheries were cool.

After 1 L of saline, his heart rate improved to 100 bpm. Routine trauma radiography revealed three rib fractures and two lumbar transverse process fractures and suspicion of a right-sided pelvic fracture. Despite apparent cardiovascular stability over the next 30 min, he again became tachycardic.

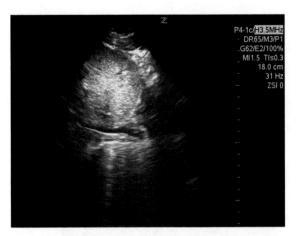

Figure 7.6 **The inferior vena cava in significant hypovolaemia.**

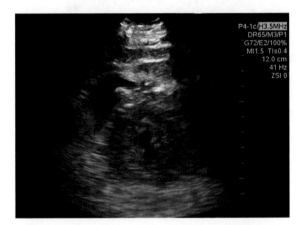

Figure 7.7 **Parasternal short axis view showing very small end-systolic dimensions, approaching papillary apposition.**

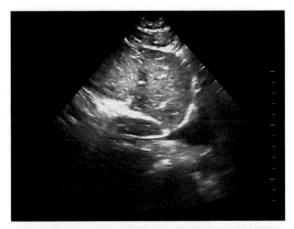

Figure 7.8 **[Video 7.1] A profoundly collapsing inferior vena cava seen from the subcostal view.**

This video is available to watch in the online video appendix.

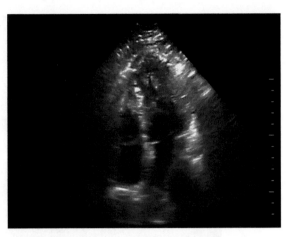

Figure 7.9 **[Video 7.2] A small hyperdynamic left ventricle with papillary muscle apposition in systole seen in the apical four-chamber view.**

This video is available to watch in the online video appendix.

Emergency echocardiography was performed with the following findings: a hyperdynamic LV with small diastolic dimensions and near papillary apposition, and an IVC dimension of 1.1 cm on expiration, with complete collapse during inspiration. These echocardiographic features are demonstrated in Figures 7.6 and 7.7, and 7.8 ⊙, and 7.9 ⊙.

A further rapid fluid bolus was administered and an urgent CT scan organized. This confirmed pelvic and transverse process fractures but also demonstrated a large retroperitoneal haematoma and suspicion of a ruptured renal artery. Further circulatory instability ensued and the abdominal girth was noted to have increased.

Further resuscitation was given with blood products and an emergency laparotomy was performed, the damaged vessel repaired, and haemostasis achieved, and the patient was extubated later that day on the intensive care unit. Repeat echocardiography following the procedure demonstrated an end-diastolic dimension of 5.1 cm and an IVC of 2.0 cm without 20% collapse on inspiration.

Fluid responsiveness

Stroke volume or flow velocity variation

Survey the potential sample points for the best available on-axis pulsed-wave Doppler cursor position for the assessment of the SV or flow velocity variation.

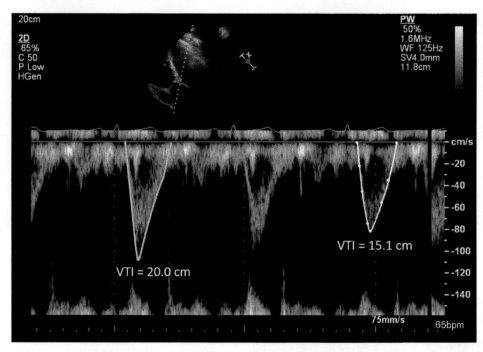

Figure 7.10 Using the flow variation sampled in the left ventricular outflow tract, this example shows a velocity time integral variation of 28%. If this patient had no spontaneous respiratory effort, this study would strongly suggest fluid responsiveness. However, if they were breathing spontaneously, it is not possible to accurately draw a conclusion about fluid responsiveness from this result.

Accurate sites for assessment include:

1. The LVOT in the apical five-chamber or three-chamber view

2. The RVOT in the right ventricular outflow view or parasternal short axis view at the pulmonary valve level.

The accepted formula for calculating flow variation is the difference between the highest and lowest flow as a percentage of the mean of the largest and smallest flow. On the assumption that the LVOT has a constant diameter, it is not necessary to actually calculate the SV and the area under the velocity–time waveform; the VTI may be used:

$$(1) \quad VTI\,variation\,(\%) = \frac{100 \times (VTI_{max} - VTI_{min})}{[(VTI_{max} + VTI_{min}) \times 0.5]}$$

Figure 7.10 illustrates a worked example.

$$(2) \quad VTI\,variation\,(\%) = \frac{100 \times (20.0 - 15.1)}{[(20.0 + 15.1) \times 0.5]}$$

$$(3) \quad SVV\,or\,VTI\,variation\,(\%) = \frac{(100 \times 4.9)}{(35.1 \times 0.5)} = 28$$

Alternatively, the peak velocity of a pulsed-wave Doppler-acquired waveform can be used in place of the VTI to good effect. Peak velocity is probably slightly less accurate than the VTI for calculation of the SVV, but a cut-off of 10–15% variation is commonly used with both VTI and peak velocity variation.

CASE STUDY

Acute pancreatitis and hypoxia: fluid deficit or excess?

A 68-year-old man was admitted with abdominal pain and malaise. He had a background of heavy alcohol use and ischaemic heart disease for which he had had percutaneous coronary intervention. He was tachycardic, with a normal blood pressure.

Imaging and an elevated amylase suggested a diagnosis of pancreatitis. There was no evidence of biliary obstruction, and excessive alcohol use was thought to be causative.

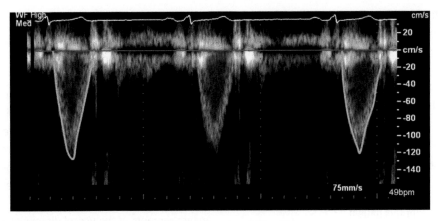

Figure 7.11 **Left ventricular outflow tract velocity time integral variation 8%.**

In view of his predicted low severity, he was admitted to the general surgical ward for ongoing management.

However, overnight his respiratory rate and oxygen requirement increased rapidly. The intensive care team was called to review due to concern that acute respiratory distress syndrome was developing after a chest radiograph showed bilateral infiltrates. On their arrival, the patient was in extremis and emergency tracheal intubation was necessary prior to transfer to the unit. Mean arterial blood pressure whilst ventilated was 55 mmHg and a noradrenaline infusion was set up.

Bedside echocardiography was performed whilst on full mechanical ventilation (including muscle relaxation). The findings were:

- Hyperdynamic left ventricular function. Mild to moderate diastolic impairment
- The RV was mildly dilated but had normal function
- Right atrial dilation. Dilated IVC with no variation through the respiratory cycle
- Flow variation across the LVOT was 8% and a passive leg raise induced an increment in SV of <5%
- B predominance was also noted on pleural ultrasound.

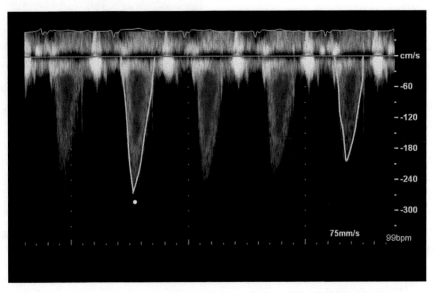

Figure 7.12 **Left ventricular outflow tract velocity time integral variation 18% after diuresis.**

It was concluded that fluid removal would be both beneficial and well tolerated. An intravenous fluid infusion was ceased and a bolus of furosemide was given, followed by an infusion. This resulted in significant diuresis and concurrent rapid weaning of oxygen concentration and ventilator pressures. The endotracheal tube was removed by the following day and the patient was managed with face-mask oxygen on intensive care for one further day. He continued to improve and was discharged home within a further week.

Figures 7.11 and 7.12 shows the LVOT VTI at two stages in the management of this patient.

Passive leg raising

TTE is an accurate measure of SV and cardiac output. Passive leg raising can then be used to measure the effect of a stressed volume load on cardiac output using the VTI as a surrogate. Use the following steps to make this assessment:

1. Assess the quality of the image of the LVOT in the apical five- and apical three-chamber views. The RVOT may also be used to make this assessment. Either the right ventricular outflow view or the parasternal short axis view at the level of the aortic valve can be used

2. Angle the probe to place the cursor line as in line as possible with the blood flow. Sample flow using pulsed-wave Doppler and freeze the view and trace the VTI envelope. Where there is visible flow variation, it is best to measure at least three waveforms and calculate a mean. This calculation is usually done automatically following tracing on newer echo platforms

3. Passively raise the patient's legs. Moving the patient should be done carefully, but fairly swiftly to achieve the effect of a fluid bolus delivered into the central circulation, whilst avoiding discomfort since a pain response might be expected to increase the cardiac output and invalidate the test. The position should be held for 90–120 s

4. Find the same view again and repeat the measurement. An increment in average VTI of >10% predicts fluid responsiveness. Return the patient to their standard position.

Inferior vena cava diameter variation

The maximum and minimum diametera of the IVC throughout the respiratory cycle in a fully ventilated patient without spontaneous respiratory effort can be measured at a point just distal to the origin of a hepatic vein, as shown in Figure 7.13. The diameter should be measured ensuring the bright edge of the vessel is seen clearly for the entire length of the respiratory cycle. If the cursor line cuts the IVC perpendicularly, then M-mode provides a convenient way of doing this. If not, then 2D should be used with point-to-point measurements of the vessel dimensions.

The IVC is viewed using the standard subxiphoid position, but good images may be obtained more laterally through a rib space and the liver. This is particularly useful where a fresh midline laparotomy wound precludes the standard view. Care should be taken to ensure the image plane is aligned with the IVC throughout the respiratory cycle, as any movement of the imaging plane to the side of the vessel will cause an apparent reduction in diameter.

In spontaneously breathing patients without positive pressure ventilation, the IVC collapsibility index is only useful close to the extremes of fluid balance. A small vessel that collapses 50% or more during inspiration suggests fluid will at least be tolerated. A dilated vessel that changes <15% with the respiratory cycle suggests that cardiac output is unlikely to increase with fluid

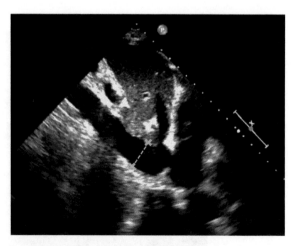

Figure 7.13 Measurement point for assessment of inferior vena cava diameter variation. This can be done using M-mode, but this necessitates the cursor line to be perpendicular to the vessel throughout the respiratory cycle.

loading and the risk of increasing extravascular lung water may be significant.

In the ventilated patient without respiratory effort, the distensibility may be expressed as a percentage in two ways:

(4) $(Dmax - Dmin) / Dmin$

5. $(Dmax - Dmin) / [0.5 \times (Dmax + Dmin)]$

(D = diameter)

The reference ranges vary according to the formula used.

For the first of these indices, a 'distensibility index' of around 18% or more predicts fluid responsiveness in a ventilated patient without respiratory effort. For the second index, 12% should be used as the approximate cut-off. Direct measurement is advised, as visual assessment of diameter variation is accurate only with the very experienced eye.

Practice point

The accuracy of using the vena cava as a mechanism for assessing fluid responsiveness is reduced by:

1. Spontaneous ventilator triggering by the patient
2. Pressure supported, as opposed to full positive pressure mechanical ventilation
3. Large tidal volumes
4. High work of breathing
5. High intra-abdominal pressures.

Fluid removal

Acutely, fluid removal may be desirable where high blood volume is suspected. Such situations include pulmonary oedema, renal impairment, and over-resuscitation. Excessive circulating volume will be revealed by findings suggesting a lack of fluid responsiveness. IVC diameter variability, SVV, or response to a passive leg raise may be used to cap fluid removal when the circulation becomes fluid-responsive once more.

Following the resuscitation phase of critical illness, most patients are left with a positive fluid balance, much of which resides in the non-vascular, non-cellular interstitial space. In time, tissue oedema will resolve as the inflammatory response fades away and intercellular connections, and therefore vascular permeability, return to a normal state. Clinicians sometimes elect to accelerate this process using diuretics or haemofiltration to assist patient progression towards extubation by removing interstitial pulmonary fluid.

This is a relatively new area of practice for critical care echocardiography. In the same way that dynamic markers may be used to make decisions about fluid administration, they have begun to be used to guide fluid removal. Lung ultrasound also has an evolving role in the diagnosis and management of fluid overload. The finding of bilateral B line predominance on imaging the lung suggests excessive extravascular lung water.

The precise method for employing echocardiography for this purpose is not yet clear, but it is important that serial assessments be made as increasing SVV of IVC variability implies a reduction in SV. Where patients have a large amount of tissue oedema, then the rate of refilling of the circulation will become apparent with repeated examination of fluid responsiveness markers and the rate of fluid removal adjusted accordingly. Frequent surveillance of both markers of clinical improvement (oxygen requirement, oedema, and fluid balance) and deleterious consequences (markers of perfusion or renal insufficiency) is vital.

Volume assessment algorithm

Although echocardiography is a powerful tool in volume assessment, no echocardiographic feature is entirely sensitive or specific, and several are unhelpfully affected by the physiology in critical illness. In addition, attaining the necessary usable images may be difficult or impossible in a significant proportion of patients.

All findings must be put in clinical context. Clearly identifying the clinical question you are asking improves pre-test probability and helps technique selection. Where conflicting findings arise, it is necessary to decide which are likely to be the most valid in that particular patient. 'Grey zone' findings, such as flow variation results on, or very close to, cut-off values, should also prompt the use of additional modalities. Where uncertainty persists, a recently adopted approach is to look at the reaction to a small, rapid bolus of fluid. As little as 100 mL is given quickly and the assessment repeated.

These algorithms take you through a clinical approach to using TTE for the assessment of volume status (Figure 7.14) and fluid responsiveness (Figure 7.15) and include prompts about clinical factors affecting the accuracy of that assessment.

Multiple choice questions

1. Echocardiographic markers with good specificity for frank hypovolaemia include:

A Velocity time integral variation of 20% in a spontaneously breathing patient

B Papillary apposition in the absence of significant left ventricular hypertrophy, vasodilatation, or inotropy

C A non-dilated inferior vena cava varying 20% in a ventilated patient

D A 15% rise in velocity time integral value 90 s after a passive leg raise

E A hyperdynamic left ventricle with a low indexed end-diastolic dimension previously in the normal range

2. Findings supporting a prediction of fluid responsiveness in a ventilated patient with no spontaneous respiratory effort include:

A A normal right ventricular end-diastolic dimension

B Inferior vena cava variability index of 20%

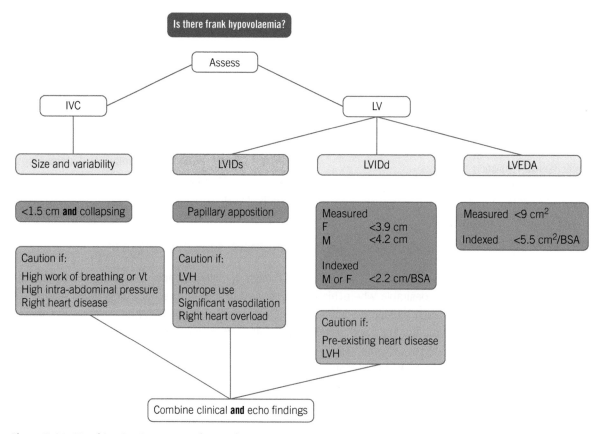

Figure 7.14 Algorithm for the echocardiographic assessment for hypovolaemia. The features suggestive of hypovolaemia are detailed here. Left ventricle internal dimension at end-systolic (dark shading) is the most validated of these measures, but all findings must be put in clinical context. IVC, inferior vena cava; LV, left ventricle; LVIDs, left ventricle internal dimension at end-systolic; LVEDA, left ventricle end-diastolic area; BSA, body surface area; LVH, left ventricular hypertrophy.

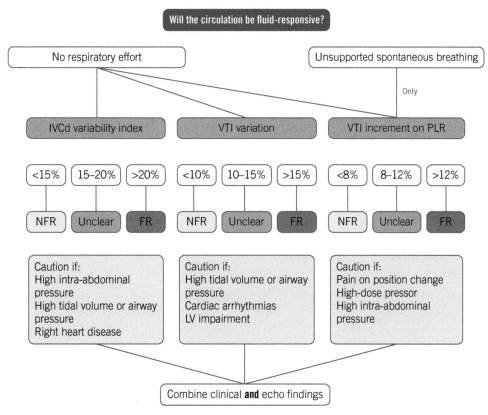

Figure 7.15 **Algorithm for the assessment of fluid responsiveness using echocardiography.** IVC variability index = (Dmax − Dmin)/0.5 × (Dmax + Dmin). NFR, fluid responsiveness unlikely; FR, fluid responsiveness predicted; IVCd, inferior vena cava diameter; VTI, velocity time integral; PLR, passive leg raising.

C Velocity time integral variation of 20%
D Velocity time integral increment of 6% after passive leg raising
E A small right atrium

3. Tolerance to volume loading is suggested by:
   A Right ventricular dilatation and minor septal flattening
   B Inferior vena cava variability of 50% in spontaneous ventilation
   C Inferior vena cava variability of 60% in mechanical ventilation with paralysis
   D Velocity time integral variation of 10% in mechanical ventilation with paralysis
   E An elevated E/e' value

4. Well-documented confounders in the assessment of velocity time integral response to passive leg raising include:
   A A tidal volume of 7 mL/kg
   B Cardiac arrhythmias

C An intra-abdominal pressure of 10 mmHg
D High work of breathing
E High-dose vasopressor use

5. When making management decisions based on echocardiographic findings:
   A Pre-test probability is of little relevance
   B Fluid responsiveness implies blood pressure responsiveness
   C As many markers as possible should be assessed
   D Visual qualitative assessment is more accurate than quantitative assessment
   E Fluid responsiveness does not imply fluid is required

For answers to multiple choice questions, please see 'Appendix 1: Answers to multiple choice questions', p. 171.

Further reading

Cecconi M, De Backer D, Antonelli M, *et al.* Consensus on circulatory shock and hemodynamic monitoring. Task Force of the European Society of Intensive Care Medicine. *Intensive Care Med* 2014; **40**: 1795–815.

Charron C, Caille V, Jardin F, Vieillard-Baron A. Echocardiographic measurement of fluid responsiveness. *Curr Opin Crit Care* 2006; **12**: 249–54.

De Backer D, Cholley BP, Slama M, Vieillard-Baron A, Vignon P (eds). *Hemodynamic monitoring using echocardiography in the critically ill.* Springer, Berlin, 2011.

De Backer D, Fagnoul D. Intensive care ultrasound: VI. Fluid responsiveness and shock assessment. *Ann Am Thorac Soc* 2014; **11**: 129–36.

Gerstle J, Shahul S, Mahmood F. Echocardiographically derived parameters of fluid responsiveness. *Int Anaesthesiol Clin* 2010; **48**: 37–44.

Mandeville J, Colebourn C. Can transthoracic echocardiography be used to predict fluid responsiveness in the critically ill patient? A systematic review. *Crit Care Res Pract* 2012; **2012**: 513480.

Marik PE, Monnet X, Teboul J-L. Hemodynamic parameters to guide fluid therapy. *Ann Intensive Care* 2011; **1**: 1.

Royse CF, Soeding PF, Blake DW. Shape and movement of the interatrial septum predicts change in pulmonary capillary wedge pressure. *Ann Thoracic Cardiovasc Surg* 2001; **7**: 79–83.

8

Field guide to critical care echocardiography

This chapter aims to merge the knowledge and techniques explored in the previous chapters and provide clinical echocardiographers with working guides for use at the bedside.

This chapter is designed around common presentations and clinical questions posed by critical care teams and includes:

1. Volume status algorithm

2. Fluid responsiveness algorithm in the ventilated and non-ventilated patient

3. An approach to the shocked, short-of-breath, and traumatized patient

4. Assessment of advanced haemodynamics

5. Decision algorithm for thrombolysis in PE

6. Guide to the echocardiographic investigation of the sick and peri-arrest obstetric patient

7. Algorithm for the echocardiographic investigation of the patient who is failing to wean from mechanical ventilation.

Every algorithm uses the following key:

- Grey/lightest box: caution

- Light blue/medium-shaded boxes: a step in the algorithm

- Blue/darkest box: emergency action required

- Bold text: equation or a calculation or a warning/ emphasis.

Volume status algorithm

Contemporary practice is now based on the prediction and assessment of fluid responsiveness since static

markers are prone to misinterpretation. Fluid responsiveness assessment is shown in the next algorithm. However, it is still important to be able to recognize the features of:

- Severe hypovolaemia

- Severe hypervolaemia, and

- To understand the derivation of the corrected flow time in order to use echocardiography and oesophageal Doppler monitoring in combination.

These key echocardiographic concepts are shown in the algorithm in Figure 8.1.

Fluid responsiveness algorithm in the ventilated and non-ventilated patient

Key concepts

- The assessment of fluid responsiveness is different in the ventilated and non-ventilated patient.

- In the non-ventilated patient, as the work of breathing goes up, so too does the cyclical reduction in flow of blood into the right heart. **This is not a reflection of fluid responsiveness. It is a result of augmented negative intrathoracic pressure at the start of normal respiration.**

- Assessment of fluid responsiveness in the fully ventilated patient is much more reliable since the work of breathing has largely been removed; therefore, cyclical changes in intravascular volume with respiration become a more accurate reflection of fluid responsiveness.

- Full pre-conditions for using SV/cardiac output/VTI/ peak velocity variation (measured at the LVOT) must

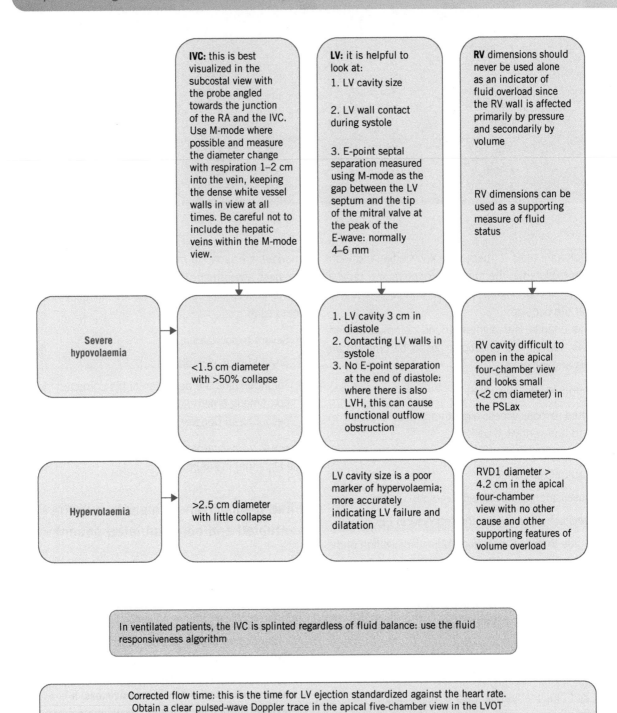

Figure 8.1 **Algorithm for the assessment of volume status.**

be met; otherwise response to a fluid bolus or passive leg raise is the only reliable mechanism of measuring fluid responsiveness using these parameters.

- Pre-conditions are given in the algorithm.
- The definition of fluid responsiveness is a 10–15% increase in cardiac output 15–30 min following the delivery of a 500-mL fluid bolus.
- If you suspect a false-negative response has been achieved, demonstrate an increase in transmitral E wave and E/A ratio with a fluid bolus, to be convinced that additional volume has impacted the central circulation adequately to measure a response.
- The algorithm is shown in Figure 8.2.

Advanced haemodynamics

Critical care echocardiography can obviate the need for invasive monitoring and is a powerful adjunct to clinical assessment of the three key circulatory compartments:

- Cardiac structure and current function: this allows the clinician to position the systolic ventricular function on the correct Starling curve and assess filling pressures
- Capacitance compartment: optimization of fluid responsiveness
- Small vessels: estimation of the SVR.

Echocardiography is unique from other cardiovascular monitors in that it combines qualitative and quantitative information: this builds a full picture of the cardiovascular status, reducing judgement errors.

Performing a full study is vital to the correct interpretation of structure and cardiovascular function. Any repeat studies required are then quick to perform and should be focused on correction of detected problems or confirmation of clinical trends.

An algorithm to guide the assessment of advanced haemodynamic parameters is shown in Figure 8.3.

An approach to the shocked, short-of-breath, or traumatized patient

This common clinical scenario requires a two-stage approach:

- Firstly, a systematic, but rapid, search for key decision-making pathology, and
- Secondly, a follow-up study when the patient has received the necessary first-line treatment to obtain complete echocardiographic information and check for treatment response.

The algorithm in Figure 8.4 shows a systematic approach to the unwell patient.

Decision algorithm for thrombolysis in pulmonary embolism

The diagnosis of a haemodynamically significant PE is based on:

- A compatible clinical history and clinical findings suggesting right heart strain, including tachycardia, right ventricular heave, and in severe cases systemic hypotension
- Echocardiography should be the first test performed where a massive or sub-massive PE is suspected. CTPA scanning is not indicated until the patient is stabilized and treated
- Thrombolysis is indicated in **massive** PE, defined as evidence of right heart strain on echocardiography and systemic hypotension where the diagnosis is most likely to be PE
- Thrombolysis in **sub-massive** PE where there is evidence of right heart strain but no systemic hypotension is more contentious, but given growing clinical appreciation of the short-term mortality risk and long-term morbidity of a sub-massive PE, current best practice supports thrombolysis where the bleeding risk is considered low

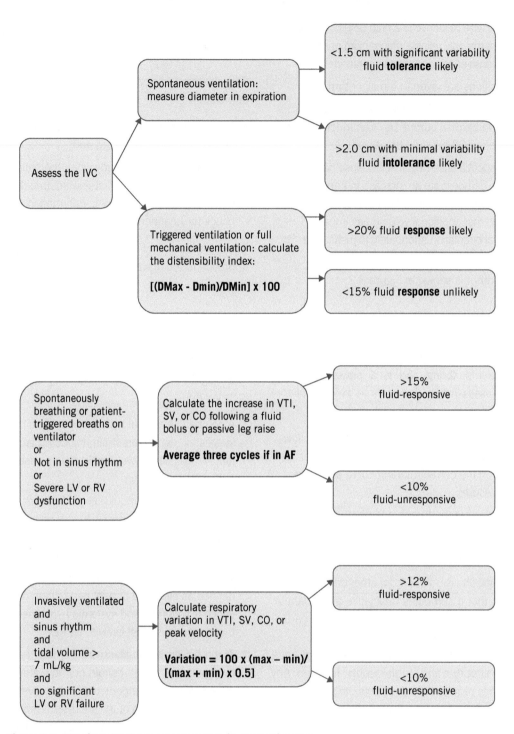

Figure 8.2 Algorithm for the assessment of fluid responsiveness.

Reproduced with kind permission from Ashley Miller and Justin Mandeville.

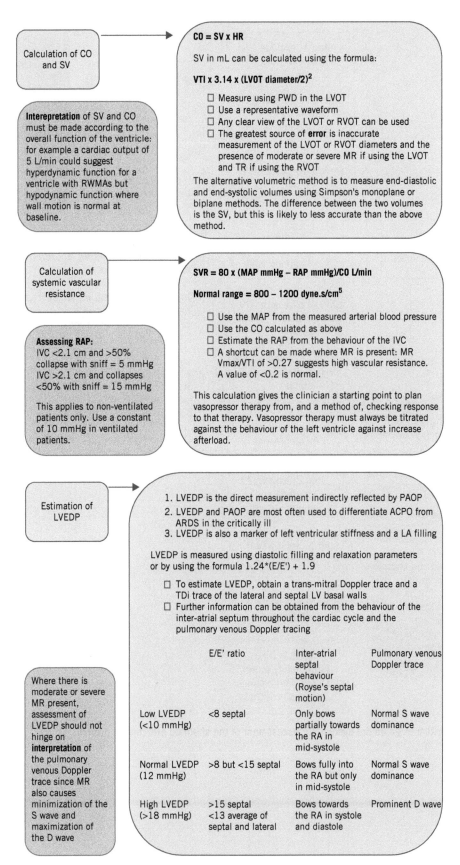

Calculation of CO and SV

CO = SV x HR

SV in mL can be calculated using the formula:

VTI x 3.14 x (LVOT diameter/2)^2

☐ Measure using PWD in the LVOT
☐ Use a representative waveform
☐ Any clear view of the LVOT or RVOT can be used
☐ The greatest source of **error** is inaccurate measurement of the LVOT or RVOT diameters and the presence of moderate or severe MR if using the LVOT and TR if using the RVOT

The alternative volumetric method is to measure end-diastolic and end-systolic volumes using Simpson's monoplane or biplane methods. The difference between the two volumes is the SV, but this is likely to less accurate than the above method.

Intererpretation of SV and CO must be made according to the overall function of the ventricle: for example a cardiac output of 5 L/min could suggest hyperdynamic function for a ventricle with RWMAs but hypodynamic function where wall motion is normal at baseline.

Calculation of systemic vascular resistance

SVR = 80 x (MAP mmHg – RAP mmHg)/CO L/min

Normal range = 800 – 1200 dyne.s/cm^5

☐ Use the MAP from the measured arterial blood pressure
☐ Use the CO calculated as above
☐ Estimate the RAP from the behaviour of the IVC
☐ A shortcut can be made where MR is present: MR Vmax/VTI of >0.27 suggests high vascular resistance. A value of <0.2 is normal.

This calculation gives the clinician a starting point to plan vasopressor therapy from, and a method of, checking response to that therapy. Vasopressor therapy must always be titrated against the behaviour of the left ventricle against increase afterload.

Assessing RAP:
IVC <2.1 cm and >50% collapse with sniff = 5 mmHg
IVC >2.1 cm and collapses <50% with sniff = 15 mmHg

This applies to non-ventilated patients only. Use a constant of 10 mmHg in ventilated patients.

Estimation of LVEDP

1. LVEDP is the direct measurement indirectly reflected by PAOP
2. LVEDP and PAOP are most often used to differentiate ACPO from ARDS in the critically ill
3. LVEDP is also a marker of left ventricular stiffness and a LA filling

LVEDP is measured using diastolic filling and relaxation parameters or by using the formula 1.24*(E/E') + 1.9

☐ To estimate LVEDP, obtain a trans-mitral Doppler trace and a TDi trace of the lateral and septal LV basal walls
☐ Further information can be obtained from the behaviour of the inter-atrial septum throughout the cardiac cycle and the pulmonary venous Doppler tracing

	E/E' ratio	Inter-atrial septal behaviour (Royse's septal motion)	Pulmonary venous Doppler trace
Low LVEDP (<10 mmHg)	<8 septal	Only bows partially towards the RA in mid-systole	Normal S wave dominance
Normal LVEDP (12 mmHg)	>8 but <15 septal	Bows fully into the RA but only in mid-systole	Normal S wave dominance
High LVEDP (>18 mmHg)	>15 septal <13 average of septal and lateral	Bows towards the RA in systole and diastole	Prominent D wave

Where there is moderate or severe MR present, assessment of LVEDP should not hinge on **interpretation** of the pulmonary venous Doppler trace since MR also causes minimization of the S wave and maximization of the D wave

Figure 8.3 Algorithm for the assessment of advanced haemodynamics.

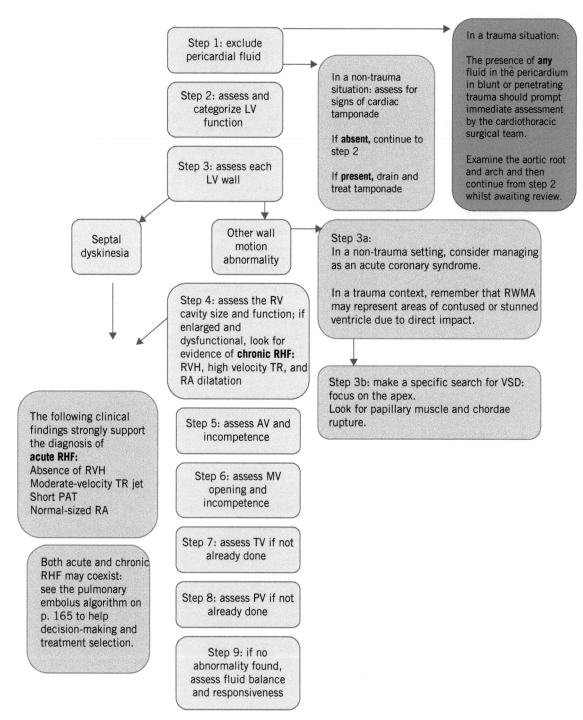

Figure 8.4 Algorithm to guide the systematic assessment of the shocked and unwell patient.

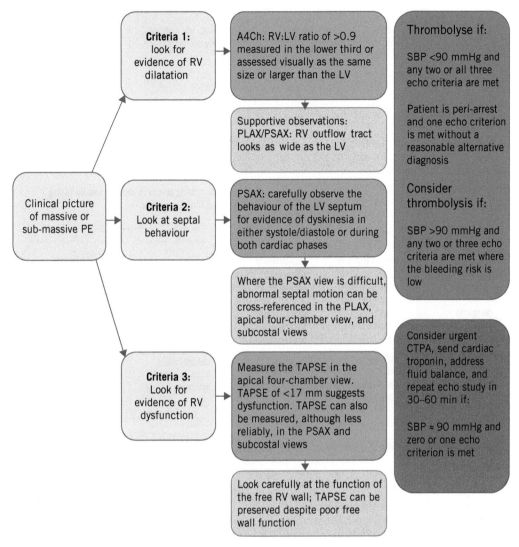

Figure 8.5 Algorithm for the assessment of the patient with a suspected acute pulmonary embolism.

- The algorithm shown in Figure 8.5 is designed to help clinicians balance the >50% mortality from a massive and sub-massive PE with the 1–2% risk of haemorrhagic stroke from thrombolysis.

- Repeat and full studies should follow, as indicated by the clinical context
- An algorithm to guide the rapid assessment of the critically unwell obstetric patient is shown in Figure 8.6.

Guide to the echocardiographic investigation of the sick and peri-arrest obstetric patient

- The clinician echocardiographer can play a vital role in reducing the time to treatment for this vulnerable population
- This algorithm is designed to get to a likely diagnosis as rapidly as possible

Echocardiographic investigation of the patient who is failing to wean from mechanical ventilation

Failed attempts at extubation and slow weaning from mechanical ventilation may reflect underlying or inter-current cardiac conditions.

- A full study is indicated.

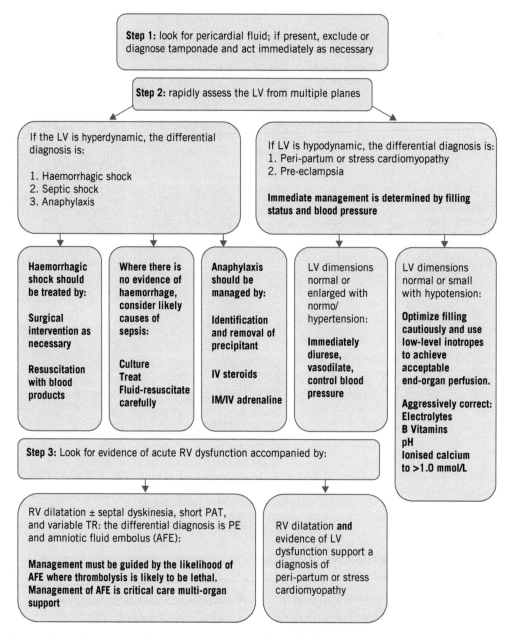

Step 1: look for pericardial fluid; if present, exclude or diagnose tamponade and act immediately as necessary

Step 2: rapidly assess the LV from multiple planes

If the LV is hyperdynamic, the differential diagnosis is:

1. Haemorrhagic shock
2. Septic shock
3. Anaphylaxis

If LV is hypodynamic, the differential diagnosis is:
1. Peri-partum or stress cardiomyopathy
2. Pre-eclampsia

Immediate management is determined by filling status and blood pressure

Haemorrhagic shock should be treated by:

Surgical intervention as necessary

Resuscitation with blood products

Where there is no evidence of haemorrhage, consider likely causes of sepsis:

Culture Treat Fluid-resuscitate carefully

Anaphylaxis should be managed by:

Identification and removal of precipitant

IV steroids

IM/IV adrenaline

LV dimensions normal or enlarged with normo/hypertension:

Immediately diurese, vasodilate, control blood pressure

LV dimensions normal or small with hypotension:

Optimize filling cautiously and use low-level inotropes to achieve acceptable end-organ perfusion.

Aggressively correct: Electrolytes B Vitamins pH Ionised calcium to >1.0 mmol/L

Step 3: Look for evidence of acute RV dysfunction accompanied by:

RV dilatation ± septal dyskinesia, short PAT, and variable TR: the differential diagnosis is PE and amniotic fluid embolus (AFE):

Management must be guided by the likelihood of AFE where thrombolysis is likely to be lethal. Management of AFE is critical care multi-organ support

RV dilatation **and** evidence of LV dysfunction support a diagnosis of peri-partum or stress cardiomyopathy

Figure 8.6 Algorithm to guide the rapid assessment of the critically unwell obstetric patient.

- Echoing whilst the patient is under 'weaning stress', for example during an SBT, is more likely to reveal any underlying cardiac abnormality such as right wall motion abnormality, AS, MR, LVOT gradient, or poor LV relaxation.

- Large pleural effusions can precipitate diastolic dysfunction and should be sought and treated.

- The algorithm shown in Figure 8.7 is designed to guide the clinician through the thought processes required during assessment of failure to wean from mechanical ventilation.

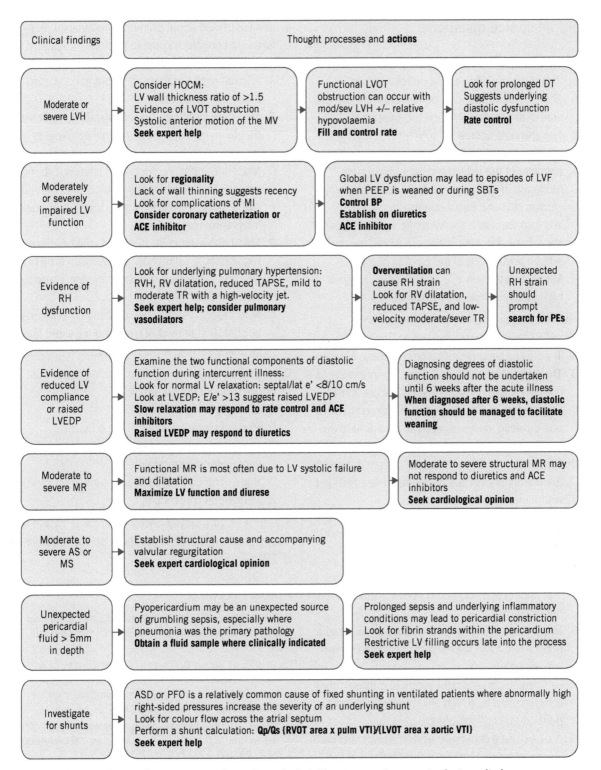

Clinical findings	Thought processes and **actions**
Moderate or severe LVH	**Consider HOCM:** LV wall thickness ratio of >1.5; Evidence of LVOT obstruction; Systolic anterior motion of the MV; **Seek expert help** → Functional LVOT obstruction can occur with mod/sev LVH +/– relative hypovolaemia **Fill and control rate** → Look for prolonged DT Suggests underlying diastolic dysfunction **Rate control**
Moderately or severely impaired LV function	Look for **regionality**; Lack of wall thinning suggests recency; Look for complications of MI; **Consider coronary catheterization or ACE inhibitor** → Global LV dysfunction may lead to episodes of LVF when PEEP is weaned or during SBTs **Control BP**; **Establish on diuretics**; **ACE inhibitor**
Evidence of RH dysfunction	Look for underlying pulmonary hypertension: RVH, RV dilatation, reduced TAPSE, mild to moderate TR with a high-velocity jet. **Seek expert help; consider pulmonary vasodilators** → **Overventilation** can cause RH strain; Look for RV dilatation, reduced TAPSE, and low-velocity moderate/sever TR → Unexpected RH strain should prompt **search for PEs**
Evidence of reduced LV compliance or raised LVEDP	Examine the two functional components of diastolic function during intercurrent illness: Look for normal LV relaxation: septal/lat e' <8/10 cm/s; Look at LVEDP: E/e' >13 suggest raised LVEDP **Slow relaxation may respond to rate control and ACE inhibitors**; **Raised LVEDP may respond to diuretics** → Diagnosing degrees of diastolic function should not be undertaken until 6 weeks after the acute illness **When diagnosed after 6 weeks, diastolic function should be managed to facilitate weaning**
Moderate to severe MR	Functional MR is most often due to LV systolic failure and dilatation **Maximize LV function and diurese** → Moderate to severe structural MR may not respond to diuretics and ACE inhibitors **Seek cardiological opinion**
Moderate to severe AS or MS	Establish structural cause and accompanying valvular regurgitation **Seek expert cardiological opinion**
Unexpected pericardial fluid > 5mm in depth	Pyopericardium may be an unexpected source of grumbling sepsis, especially where pneumonia was the primary pathology **Obtain a fluid sample where clinically indicated** → Prolonged sepsis and underlying inflammatory conditions may lead to pericardial constriction; Look for fibrin strands within the pericardium; Restrictive LV filling occurs late into the process **Seek expert help**
Investigate for shunts	ASD or PFO is a relatively common cause of fixed shunting in ventilated patients where abnormally high right-sided pressures increase the severity of an underlying shunt; Look for colour flow across the atrial septum; Perform a shunt calculation: **Qp/Qs {RVOT area x pulm VTI}/{LVOT area x aortic VTI}** **Seek expert help**

Figure 8.7 Echocardiographic assessment of a patient who is failing to wean from mechanical ventilation.

Multiple choice questions

1. The following statements regarding advanced echocardiographic haemodynamics are true:
   A The cardiac output can be calculated using the area of the aortic valve and the heart rate
   B The greatest source of error in calculating the cardiac output is in the measurement of the diameter of the left ventricular outflow tract
   C Moderate mitral regurgitation does not affect cardiac output measurement accuracy
   D You can calculate the systemic vascular resistance from the right atrial pressure, the mean arterial pressure, and the cardiac output
   E Mitral regurgitation V_{max} / VTI of >0.1 suggests a high systemic vascular resistance

2. The following are true of left ventricular end-diastolic pressure measurements in the critically ill:
   A They are an accurate reflection of diastolic function
   B The left ventricular end-diastolic pressure is equivalent to the PAOP or left atrial pressure
   C E/E' septum of 5 and prominent pulmonary venous diastolic waves suggest a normal left ventricular end-diastolic pressure
   D E/E' lateral of 15 and diastolic dominance in the pulmonary venous waves suggest a high left ventricular end-diastolic pressure
   E The inter-atrial septum normally bows one way throughout the cardiac cycle

3. In the unwell obstetric patient, the following statements are true:
   A The finding of mild left ventricular impairment is not significant
   B Mild mitral regurgitation should be considered a normal finding in the context of a hyperdynamic left ventricle
   C Left ventricular and right ventricular impairment accompanied by a high blood pressure suggests peripartum cardiomyopathy
   D A slit-like right ventricular and left ventricular wall kissing suggests a major haemorrhage is likely
   E A normal-sized right ventricle and a hyperdynamic left ventricle rule out the diagnosis of major haemorrhage

4. In a suspected acute pulmonary embolism, the following echocardiographic findings indicate thrombolysis is immediately required:
   A Normal right heart size and pulmonary acceleration time of 90 ms
   B Moderate right ventricular dilatation, right ventricular hypertrophy, and normal tricuspid annular plane systolic excursion
   C Moderate right ventricular dilatation, no right ventricular hypertrophy, tricuspid annular plane systolic excursion of 1.1 cm, and bowed interventricular septum
   D Mild right ventricular dilatation, mild pulmonary regurgitation, pulmonary acceleration time of 80 ms, and borderline tricuspid annular plane systolic excursion
   E Mild right ventricular dilatation, pulmonary acceleration time of 60 ms, and tricuspid annular plane systolic excursion of 1.2 cm

5. The following are recognized cardiac causes of failure to wean from a ventilator:
   A Mild mitral regurgitation
   B Pseudonormal diastolic filling pattern
   C Moderate aortic regurgitation with moderate left ventricular dysfunction
   D Right ventricular systolic pressure of 55 mmHg
   E Pericardial constriction

For answers to multiple choice questions, please see 'Appendix 1: Answers to multiple choice questions', p. 171.

Further reading

Castillo C, Tapson VF. Right ventricular responses to massive and submassive pulmonary embolism. *Cardiol Clin* 2012; **30**: 233–41.

Cecconi M, De Backer D, Antonelli M, *et al.* Concensus on circulatory shock and haemodynamic monitoring. Task force of the European Society of Intensive Care Medicine. *Intensive Care Med* 2014; **40**: 1795–815.

Dennis AT. Transthoracic echocardiography in obstetric anaesthesia and obstetric critical illness. *Int J Obstet Anesth* 2011; **20**: 160–8.

Mandeville J, Colebourn C. Can transthoracic echocardiography be used to predict fluid responsiveness in the critically ill patient? A systematic review. *Crit Care Res Pract* 2012; **2012**: 513480.

Meyer G, Vicaut E, Danays T. Fibrinolysis for patients with intermediate-risk pulmonary embolism. *N Engl J Med* 2014; **370**: 1402–11.

Morris CGT, Burn SA, Richards SB. Modern protective ventilation strategies: impact upon the right heart. *JICS* 2014; **15**: 28–33.

Moschietto S, Doyen D, Grech L, Dellamonica J, Hyvernat H, Bernardin G. Transthoracic echocardiography with Doppler tissue imaging predicts weaning failure from mechanical ventilation: evolution of the left ventricle relaxation rate during a spontaneous breathing trial is the key factor in weaning outcome. *Crit Care* 2012; **16**: R81.

Appendix 1
Answers to multiple choice questions

Chapter 2

1. FTFTF
2. TFFTF
3. FTFTT
4. FTTTF
5. FTFFF

Chapter 3

1. FFFFT
2. TTTTF
3. FFTTF
4. FTTFT
5. TTTTF

Chapter 4

1. TFFFT
2. FTFFT
3. TTFTT
4. TFTFT
5. FFTTF

Chapter 5

1. TFTFT
2. FFFTT
3. FTTFF
4. FTFFF
5. FFFFT

Chapter 6

1. FTFFT
2. FFTFT
3. FTTFT
4. TTTTT
5. TTTTF

Chapter 7

1. FTFFT
2. FTTFT
3. FTTFF
4. FFFTT
5. FFTFT

Chapter 8

1. FTFTF
2. FTFTF
3. FTFTF
4. FFTFT
5. FTTTT

Index

Tables and figures are indicated by an italic *t* and *f* following the page number.